What Others Are Saying

"Jennie Johnson's book likely saved my life. Please read and give to everyone you care about and want around for a long time. My only regret is that she didn't write it ten years ago to save my own mother. A must read."

—Debra Benton, internationally known speaker, executive coach consultant, best selling author including her recent release, *The CEO Difference* (McGraw-Hill)

"Johnson gives a powerful, solution-based approach for tackling the root causes of heart attacks and strokes. These small changes don't have to involve willpower or begging others to help. Many of her insightful solutions simply require a few adjustments to what people are already doing. What is also distinguishing about this book is that it focuses on the importance of gratitude—gratitude for each healthy day, the people in our lives, and the potential of our life. In the end, it not only strives to increase the days in our life, but to also increase the life in our days."

—Brian Wansink, PhD, author of the bestselling book
Mindless Eating and recent release *Slim By Design*,
Director of the Cornell Food and Brand Lab,
appointed by the White House in 2007 as the
USDA Executive Director in charge of the
Food Pyramid and dietary guidelines

"Jennie Johnson presents an engaging combination of education and personal and professional examples that can inspire readers to progress from contemplating changing to taking effective action to enhance their heart and their health."

—James Prochaska, PhD, Director, Cancer Prevention Research Center, author of *Changing for Good* (Stages of Change Theory)

"A wealth of critical, up to date information and practical tips. Jennie Johnson's book will empower you with the tools you need to keep you healthy-all told in a very personal style, truly from the heart. I highly recommend it."

—Stephen Devries, MD, FACC Executive Director, Gaples Institute for Integrative Cardiology, author of *What Your Doctor May Not Tell You About Cholesterol*

"Dr. Johnson's book is a fabulous treatise on heart disease, stroke and risk factors. She does a great job at detailing the critical issues with a practical, informative and comprehensive voice. This is a great read for those with heart disease or simply those at increased risk. Patients and practitioners alike will find her sage advice essential to their behavior change programs. A great easy read."

—Vincent Bufalino MD, Senior Vice President, Cardiovascular Institute Advocate Healthcare, Served in key national and international leadership roles within the American Heart Association (AHA), received numerous awards, Past AHA Physician of the Year, named multiple times to "Top Doctors in Chicago" and around the nation

"Jennie Johnson's book is for anyone who wants to avoid having a heart attack or stroke. She provides a roadmap of practical, realistic tips that anyone can do to live a healthier life. Her writing style and stories simplify complex medical information and answers questions you may have been too embarrassed to ask. Even after 30+ years as a nurse, I learned so much!"

—LeAnn Thieman, *New York Times* best-selling author of *Chicken Soup for the Nurses Soul* and *SelfCare for HealthCare*

"Please read this book. It will give you and your loved ones wisdom and practical tips to promote longevity. No one should live miserably with the after effects of a stroke or heart attack. Reduce your risk by living and eating better and following the guidelines in Jennie Johnson's book. Well written, High Five!!!"

—Michael Trantow DDS

"Dr. Johnson has truly captured the essence of knowledge that is necessary for those living with or at risk for heart disease. She presents wise recommendations for making changes in behavior that will translate into lifesaving endeavors. I will certainly recommend Dr. Johnson's book for my patients."

—Lynne T. Braun, PhD, CNP, Nurse Practitioner and Professor of Nursing, Rush University College of Nursing and University Cardiologists

"Wake Up Call 911: It's Time to Reduce Your Risk for a Heart Attack and Stroke," provides a great guideline for patients to navigate the increasingly complex world of healthcare and cardiovascular disease (CVD). Jennie's book can be the first step for all of us to begin making those changes, large or small, in order to reduce our risk factors. I especially appreciated inclusion of personal experiences and the examples of celebrities with CVD. I feel those stories bring home the point of the insidious nature in which CVD can negatively effect your health and the importance of routine healthcare. This will be recommended reading for all of my dental patients."

—David L. Carlson DDS, Mentor at Kois Center for Advanced Dentistry through Science in Seattle, Washington, named as "one of the 40 finest dentists in the Chicago area" by *Chicago Magazine*

"This comprehensive, straightforward book is indispensible for anyone seeking to reduce cardiovascular risk. Jennie Johnson uses the latest clinical guidelines and her own firsthand experiences to offer inspiration, guidance, and practical strategies for living a heart-healthy lifestyle. A *must read* for all."

—Meg Gulanick, PhD, APRN, Professor Emeritus and Past Director of the Cardiac Disease Management Program, Marcella Niehoff School of Nursing, Loyola University Chicago

"This is a concisely written and very readable book to help patients manage cardiovascular risk. It is remarkably comprehensive as it presents a wide array of complex topics and makes them understandable."

—Donald R. Chisholm, MD, AAFP

"If there is one book any average adult, regardless of age, should read about personal health and one's heart it is this book. I was actively working out and losing weight before my heart attack at age forty seven but my eating habit was what I would now consider to have been reckless, at best, after reading this book. I am sure this book will benefit you as it did me, read this book and you will find out for yourself."

—Neil Oliver, An average American

"Jennie Johnson's book is a treasure trove of helpful information for those wanting to enjoy a long and active life. Jennie answers virtually every question one might have about good health and exercise. Since God has given us only one body while here on earth, this book is a must read for those wanting to take care of this gift from Him."

—Pastor Neil Bloom, Shepherd of the Hills Lutheran Church, Rathdrum, Idaho

WAKE UP CALL

911

WAKE UP CALL
911

*It's Time To Reduce Your Risk For A
Heart Attack And Stroke*

JENNIE E. JOHNSON, RN-BC, PhD

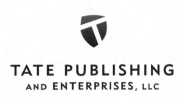

TATE PUBLISHING
AND ENTERPRISES, LLC

Published by Tate Publishing & Enterprises, LLC
127 E. Trade Center Terrace | Mustang, Oklahoma 73064 USA
1.888.361.9473 | www.tatepublishing.com

Tate Publishing is committed to excellence in the publishing industry. The company reflects the philosophy established by the founders, based on Psalm 68:11,
"The Lord gave the word and great was the company of those who published it."

Book design copyright © 2015 by Tate Publishing, LLC. All rights reserved.
Cover design by Charito Sim
Interior design by Mary Jean Archival

Published in the United States of America

ISBN: 978-1-68028-229-0
1. Health & Fitness / Diseases / Heart
2. Medical / Cardiology
15.03.25

This book is dedicated to the following people:

My husband, John, for your love and support
throughout this entire project.

My children and grandchildren who
bring so much joy to my life.

My mothers, Ilene and Ellen.

The nurses, doctors, and patients who taught me so much about
helping patients to overcome difficult health challenges.

My father, who died too young from a heart attack
at forty-six years old.

Medical Disclaimer

The goal of this book is to provide the reader with "easy to understand" information about the risk factors for heart disease. It is "not" intended to take the place of the medical advice from your healthcare provider.

Professional Disclosure

I am a co-owner of the business Living for a Healthy Heart, LLC, which provides lifestyle counseling to patients and public speaking to the community and medical audiences.

I have nothing else to disclose and no relationship with any of the pharmaceutical or technology products described within this book.

Contents

Introduction: Who Should Read This Book? 15

1 Heart Attack and Stroke Basics 19

2 Are You at Risk? 37

3 Cholesterol: The Good, the Bad, End the Confusion 55

4 High Blood Pressure: The Silent Killer 79

5 The Danger from Diabetes 103

6 The Battle of the Bulge 125

7 Strategies to Help End a Tobacco Habit 169

8 Physical Activity: Use It or Lose It 199

9 Controlling Your Response to Life's Stressors 227

10 Overcoming the Barriers to Change 241

11 Working with Your Healthcare Provider 261

12 Research and Web Sites You Can Trust 271

13 A Word to Healthcare Providers 285

14 Closing Thoughts 307

About My Services 313

About the Author 317

Acknowledgments 319

Appendix 325

Reference 333

Index 369

Introduction: Who Should Read This Book?

If you have been told by your healthcare provider that your current lifestyle increases your risk for a heart attack or stroke, this book is for you. Although fear of the health threat is heightened, changing behavior remains much easier said than done. Whether you are confused about where to begin or need help sticking with the changes that you are making, this book is for you. Even if you don't think that your lifestyle needs to change, this book will help you understand why your healthcare provider thinks it is important for you to change.

I wrote this book for an audience unfamiliar with medical jargon. It is written in simple everyday language by an experienced nurse who counseled hundreds of patients to move toward a healthier life. In addition, healthcare providers mean well, but oftentimes suggest changes that are too unrealistic for most people to follow. People stick with it for a few days but then become discouraged and quit. The failure leads to a downward spiral of destructive emotions that often increase harmful behaviors.

My goal is to meet you at your own level and, when you're ready, to help you make very simple realistic changes that fit into your everyday life. Brian Wansink[1], a noted nutrition researcher, said in his book *Mindless Eating*, "The best diet is the one you don't know that you're on." This philosophy applies to all types of behaviors. Small steps build confidence so that you can successfully change your behavior and maintain it.

The chapters of this book are designed to identify the major problems that increase risk for a heart attack or stroke: abnormal cholesterol, high blood pressure, diabetes, smoking, unhealthy eating, inactivity, excess weight, and stress. By taking care of your heart, you will improve your overall health and reduce your risk for cancer. Each chapter stands alone as a resource; however, the book may be read in its entirety. My goal is to help you change the behaviors that you want to change, not the ones that I think that you should change.

If you are a healthcare provider, this book may help you learn skills to facilitate better patient communication, understanding, and motivation for behavior change. Speaking in complex medical jargon only leads to confusion and frustration. Behavioral change is a complex process and requires small steps to help patients attain success. This book will provide you with insight into the latest research of "what works" in helping patients change harmful behaviors. In addition, the upcoming changes in health care policies will place great demands on practitioners to demonstrate positive behavior change outcomes. This book will assist you in patient approaches that are more effective.

My background is in cardiology. I have counseled hundreds of patients regarding lifestyle changes following cardiac testing and have cared for many patients following a heart attack and stroke in the hospital setting. I graduated with a PhD in nursing from Loyola University in Chicago in 2012 and studied motivation to change harmful behaviors. I wanted to explore the differences between those who were able to change harmful behaviors from those who failed. What strategies worked?

My approach is unique from most books that have been written on this topic because I include information from the medical world and from psychology. It is my goal to help you connect the dots between your actions and the harm to your health. I will help you overcome personal barriers and assist with simple steps that will enable you to succeed. For additional information on my services, philosophy, and credentials you may visit my Web site at www.living4ahealthyheart.com.

This book is dedicated to my father who died of a massive heart attack in 1977. He was only forty-six years old. His sudden untimely death has fueled my desire to prevent others from similar fates. Science has learned a great deal about detecting those at risk and intervening before they become a statistic, but heart disease remains the number 1 killer. Far too many adults continue to engage in behaviors that hurt their hearts and increase their risk for a catastrophic event.

Perhaps you are reading this book because someone close to you suffered a heart attack or stroke or your healthcare provider is concerned about your personal health. Regardless, fear can be a powerful motivator. Hopefully, this book will serve as your wake-up call that it is time to make a change toward a healthier life: more importantly, how you can do it. Benjamin Franklin's words are still powerful today: "An ounce of prevention is worth a pound of cure." So turn the page and let your journey begin, as you read about how heart disease and strokes develop and the small changes that you can make in attitude and behavior to reduce your risk.

Inaction breeds doubt and fear. Action breeds confidence and courage. If you want to conquer fear, do not sit home and think about it. Go out and get busy.

—Interpersonal Relationship Expert, Dale Carnegie

1

Heart Attack and Stroke Basics

No matter how motivated you are to change your bad habits, it is important to understand the basics of how harmful behaviors increase your risk for heart disease. The risk factors for a heart attack and stroke are the same because they are caused by the same disease process. Reducing your risk for a heart attack will also reduce your risk for a stroke. The medical term is cardiovascular disease. "Cardio" is a Latin term for "heart" and "vascular" refers to "vessels."[1] A heart attack or stroke is the result of a disease of the vessels, primarily those arteries that surround your heart and are within your brain. I begin by explaining how the heart works and why it is important to keep your arteries healthy.

How Your Heart Works

Your heart is a small muscular organ about the size of your fist that has a very important job. It pumps oxygenated nutrient-rich blood from the lungs to the rest of the body. The body needs the oxygen to make energy, to keep the cells and organs alive and working. Once the oxygen is removed from the blood, the heart pumps the blood back to the lungs where it picks up oxygen and repeats the cycle. This pumping occurs 50 to 100 times each minute over your lifetime. Think of the arteries (with oxygen) and the veins (without oxygen) as the pipes that make up this vascular roadway and keep the body working properly. A blockage leads to a roadblock in this system. Blockages in the arteries are more severe because they prevent oxygen from getting to the organs downstream.

Tourniquet Example

I often use the following example to illustrate what happens when the blood supply of oxygen is cut off. Think about what would happen if you put a tourniquet or tight rubber band around your lower right arm and left it. The tourniquet prevents oxygenated blood from getting to the tissues below the blockage. At first, you would notice a tingling sensation below the tourniquet due to the blockage. Your brain is telling you that something is wrong and you need to make a change to fix it. After a few minutes, the numbness would turn to pain. Your brain is screaming at you to release the tourniquet so that oxygenated blood can pass through. As time goes on and oxygen continues to be deprived below the tourniquet, the lower arm will turn black and die. Whenever oxygen is deprived, the tissues below the blockage dies. Your arteries must remain open to carry vital oxygen to all of the tissues of the body.

Your heart is like any other organ in the body: it also needs a supply of oxygen in order to work. The arteries that supply oxygen to the heart are called coronary arteries. Coronary is a Latin term that means "heart."[1] The coronary arteries are spaghetti-sized and surround the outside of the heart. They supply oxygen to the heart muscle so that it can keep pumping oxygen to the rest of the body. The heart works best when the arteries are wide open, getting as much oxygen as it needs.

Coronary Arteries Supply Oxygen to the Heart

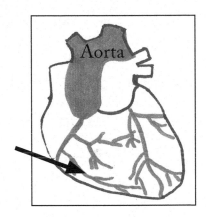

The aorta is about one inch in diameter and is the largest artery. It pumps oxygenated blood out to the rest of the body. In comparison, the spaghetti-sized coronary arteries are much smaller and supply oxygenated blood to the heart muscle. Some people get confused as to the location of a heart attack and think that it occurs when the aorta ruptures. A heart attack is caused by a blockage in one of the smaller coronary arteries that surround the heart, not by blockage of the aorta. You can see why the smaller coronary arteries would become blocked more easily than the much larger aorta.

If a blockage occurs high in the top part of the heart, it will block off oxygen to everything below it (like the tourniquet example). Most of the heart will suddenly stop working. It often results in a massive heart attack that may lead to sudden death and is also known as the widow-maker. When you hear of someone dying from a sudden heart attack, they most likely had a blockage near the top part of the heart that knocked out the entire heart's ability to pump. Conversely, if the blockage is low in the heart, there isn't as much heart muscle downstream to be altered, resulting in much less damage. This type of blockage is often called a mild heart attack. Arteries also feed oxygen to the brain. A stroke is caused by blocked arteries as well, but they are located in the brain. Just like the tourniquet example, a blockage in the heart or brain results in abnormal symptoms to warn you that something is wrong.

The Symptoms of a Heart Attack

Having a heart attack is a very scary event! It is frightening for the victim, the family, and bystanders. Unfortunately, in many cases, it may lead to death. Wherever the blockage occurs, everything downstream is impaired. The heart muscle needs oxygen to work, and it gets oxygen from the coronary arteries. Symptoms generally occur immediately when oxygen is deprived from an area in the heart. People may experience as few as one symptom or many as they vary greatly between individuals and are different between men and women. Cardiac pain is characterized by a new unusual discomfort or pain that occurs anywhere between the chin down to the navel. It can move out into the arms, up the neck, into the back, or in the teeth. Some have described the discomfort as mild while others have said, "It feels like an elephant is sitting on my chest." Women often lack these classic chest pain type symptoms but complain of unusual fatigue, nausea, or shortness of breath. Some of my patients experienced heartburn that would not go away.

Heart Attack Warning Signs
Burning, heaviness, pressure, tightness or squeezing sensation in chest.
Discomfort in jaw, shoulder, back, between the shoulder blades or down the arm.
Shortness of breath.
Fatigue, lightheadedness or weakness.
Nausea, indigestion, fatigue.
*American Heart Association

"If you or anyone around you begins to experience any of these symptoms, seek immediate medical help and call 911."[2] A heart attack even with mild symptoms can worsen and deteriorate very quickly. When the heart muscle is suddenly deprived of oxygen, a lethal heart rhythm may occur that results in death within a few minutes. A defibrillator and medical care is needed to reverse the deadly situation.

Treatment of a Heart Attack

Outside of Hospital Treatment

The first treatment that the paramedics will provide is to start oxygen for you to breathe that will increase levels in the area of the blocked artery. The area below the blockage is dying so this extra amount helps. Patients are also given aspirin to prevent the platelets from sticking together. A chewable aspirin gets into the blood faster. Normally, platelets move to an area of injury to prevent bleeding. During a heart attack, the clumping of platelets makes the blockage worse. An electrocardiogram (EKG) is applied to monitor the heart's electrical activity and locate the damaged region. The electrical activity is altered when the heart is deprived of oxygen. This may cause the heart muscle to fibrillate (quiver) and blood cannot pump effectively to the brain or vital organs. There is no pulse or blood pressure. Death quickly follows. Shocking the heart with electricity can reboot the system, and it can get the heart rhythm back to normal. Paramedics can do this with a defibrillator. However, Automatic External Defibrillator (AED) units are available for people without medical training to do the same thing. This emergency procedure can save a life. An intravenous (IV) needle is inserted to provide life-saving medications. The patient is then transported immediately to the nearest hospital. It is vital to receive medical care as soon as possible to prevent permanent damage.

Unfortunately, far too many patients ignore mild symptoms and avoid treatment. People may not want to believe that the pain or discomfort is from a heart attack. Denial that a heart attack is happening is a major barrier to receiving medical care and may result in irreversible consequences. A damaged weakened heart limits your ability to perform the activities of everyday life. There are many treatment options to open clogged arteries and return the flow of oxygen before permanent damage occurs. If you, a loved one, or a coworker experiences any of the heart attack symptoms, seek help! It is better to be safe than sorry. Time is truly of the essence.

Hospital Treatment

Once in the hospital, tests are done to determine the location of the blockage and the severity of the cardiac event. When the cardiac muscle is damaged from a lack of oxygen, enzymes are released. The timing and amount of the enzyme release is measured to determine the extent of the damage. A higher number generally indicates more damage. Patients are taken to a catheterization lab to visually look for the blocked artery.

Angiogram or Cardiac Catheterization

A cardiac catheterization involves placing a catheter or long hollow tube in the femoral artery of the groin and threading it up into the aorta. A dye is injected while the cardiologist watches how the dye travels through the coronary arteries around the heart. The dye will stop flowing if a clogged vessel is present. The cardiologist can determine the degree of blockage based on the flow of dye.

Usually the blocked artery can be treated by inflating a small balloon inside the artery (angioplasty). The artery is kept open by the placement of a stent inside the vessel. A stent is a metal corkscrew device that is placed within the artery to basically prop the artery open. The stent is coated with a medication to prevent blood cells from clogging the metal components of the stent.

Coronary Artery Bypass Grafting

Coronary artery bypass surgery (CABG) is used when the blockage is located in an area that is difficult to reach with angioplasty. A vein is removed from the leg and attached above and below the blocked artery, thus bypassing the blockage to return blood flow to the heart. The recovery is longer because it is a major operation and complications are more common. The surgeon makes a long incision down the chest to be able to visualize the blocked artery. The heart is stopped and the blood supply is shunted into a machine during the procedure. Pain, lung complications, and infection delay recovery. The recovery time from an angioplasty/stent placement takes a few days while a bypass operation takes several weeks. David Letterman and Regis Philbin are examples of celebrities who underwent this procedure.

Cardiac Rehabilitation

Cardiac rehab is a key component to recovery from a heart attack no matter what type of treatment was needed. Some patients believe that the heart problem was fixed and will not occur again. If you are someone who had an angioplasty, stent placed, or heart bypass operation, you have heart disease and will have it for the rest of your life. Just because one blockage was fixed does not mean that another one will not occur. You must make changes to keep the disease from getting worse as you get older. You now are at greater risk for another heart attack or stroke.

Cardiac rehab nurses and exercise physiologists assist patients in returning to as normal a life as possible following the cardiac event. Patients are monitored while exercising. Nurses and exercise physiologists educate patients on ways to reduce progression of the underlying plaque disease. The goal of cardiac rehab is to provide patients with confidence to return to a more active, healthier life without fear of another heart attack.[3]

I am a big supporter of cardiac rehab! I think that if you can exercise in the protected hospital environment, you will feel more confident to return to activity after your cardiac event. Any problems encountered while you exercise during cardiac rehab are immediately conveyed to the cardiologist. You also learn how to take better care of your body and work with your cardiologist to prevent another event.

A Word to Loved Ones about CPR

I believe that everyone should learn cardiopulmonary resuscitation (CPR) skills. You never know when you may be called upon to save someone's life. CPR involves learning how to get the heart pumping and the lungs providing oxygen to the tissues of the body. Without oxygen, people die within minutes. You will also learn how to use an AED defibrillator and how to help a choking victim. Pediatric (child and infant) CPR is also covered. So do not delay. Contact your local hospital, the American Heart Association (www.americanheart.org), the American Red Cross (www.redcross.org), or www.learncpr.org for the next class. The life you save might be one of your loved ones. Being knowledgeable about CPR is especially important if your loved one had a heart attack or stroke. They are at greater risk for a second event.

The Symptoms of a Stroke

The very same process of plaque build-up in the heart arteries occurs within the arteries of the brain. A blocked artery in the brain leads to a loss of oxygen to the area of the brain downstream from the blockage.

Blood Flow in the Brain

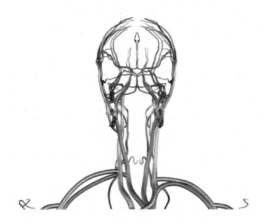

A blocked artery in the brain alters brain function. Symptoms may include numbness, pain, or headache. You may have trouble thinking, remembering, or speaking. Your face may be droopy or you are suddenly unable to move a limb. "If you experience any of these symptoms, call 911 immediately."[4]

(FAST) Stroke Warning Signs
Face Drooping: Does one side of the face droop or is it numb? Ask the person to smile. Is the person's smile uneven?
Arm Weakness: Is one arm weak or numb? Ask the person to raise both arms. Does one arm drift downward?
Speech Difficulty: Is speech slurred? Is the person unable to speak or hard to understand? Ask the person to repeat a simple sentence like, "The sky is blue." Is the sentence repeated correctly?
Time to call 911: If someone shows any of these symptoms, even if the symptoms go away, call 911 and get the person to the hospital immediately. Check the time so you'll know when the first symptoms appeared.
*American Stroke Association

I tell people that if you notice sudden symptoms on one side of your head or body more so than on the other side, call 911 immediately! It is especially important if you have a family history of stroke or heart disease. Note the exact time that the symptoms began. The medical team will want to make decisions about treatment. The sooner treatment begins, the better chance of recovery.

Patients with a history of a transient ischemic attack (TIA) are at much higher risk for a permanent stroke. A TIA is caused by a temporary clogged artery and may persist for up to twenty-four hours but often last for less than five minutes. It is a warning sign that something may be abnormal within the arteries of the brain. The next occurrence may be a full-fledge stroke.

If you have been diagnosed with a very irregular heartbeat called atrial fibrillation, you are at great risk for a stroke as well. During atrial fibrillation, blood pools in the upper part of the heart. This pooled blood can form clots. The blood clots can then be pumped out of the heart and travel into the brain or the lung, which causes a very dangerous medical emergency. In the brain, it can cause a stroke, and in the lung, a life-threatening breathing problem.

Coumadin (warfarin)[5] is a blood thinner that is often prescribed to prevent the clots from forming, but many people are reluctant to take the medication. It requires frequent blood tests to ensure that the level of thinness/thickness is just right. It takes about four days to get the blood thinned and then four days for the drug to leave your system if bleeding occurs. Foods high in Vitamin K (spinach, cabbage, potatoes, nuts, etc.) make the blood stickier and blood clots will form more easily. The Coumadin dose may need adjustment. People have to watch their diet to maintain a consistent blood thinner level. If your doctor wants you to take this medication, it is to save your life from a dangerous complication. There are other medications to thin the blood as well. Healthcare providers make decisions about which medication is best for each individual situation.

Treatment of a Stroke

As with a heart attack, many people experience mild stroke symptoms and may decide to postpone medical care, calling their healthcare provider the next day. Do not think this way! Time is life-saving in stroke, and early treatment can prevent lifelong disability. There is a clot-dissolving medication called tissue plasminogen activators (TPA) that may reverse the blockage, but it must be given within three hours of the first symptoms.[6] You must know exactly when your first stroke symptom appeared and the clock starts ticking. Not everyone can take TPA as it may cause bleeding, but few patients are given the option because they arrive at the hospital too late for the medication to work.[6] It is important to call 911 to start medical treatment for a stroke as soon as possible. When you get to the hospital, a CT scan of your brain is done immediately. The medical team will want to determine the type of stroke that you may be having. Is it a bleeding stroke or a clotting stroke? The two types of strokes are treated completely differently.

A bleeding artery causes about 13 percent of all strokes.[6] Treatment may involve observation or surgery to stop the bleeding and repair the damage. This type of stroke would not be treated with TPA, which would increase the bleeding and make the stroke worse. Some type of clotting problem causes about 87 percent of the other strokes.[6] A clot may travel from some other part of the body and reach the brain or a piece of the plaque can break off and block the artery as well. The clot needs to be dissolved and the artery opened up with the TPA medication if at all possible. It is vital that the medical team determine what type of stroke that you are having and get you the appropriate care before permanent damage occurs. Even with mild symptoms, you need to get to the hospital *immediately*! The longer the problem continues, the more damage to the brain. The new campaign from the American Heart Association and the American Stroke Association is "time is brain" to remind you to seek treatment *fast*!

Complications from a Stroke

A stroke is a very debilitating disease. The location of the blockage determines the extent and limitation of normal function. Some stroke victims are able to think clearly but not able to speak while others may lose vision. The muscles of the throat may be impaired, causing chronic choking of food resulting in lung infections. Feeding tubes are inserted to prevent further complications. A paralyzed arm or leg is especially devastating and interferes with mobility. Quality of life is profoundly impaired. Depression is a common side effect. The actor Kirk Douglas is a good example of the ramifications of a stroke. Once vibrant and active, he suffers with impaired speech. Eliminating risk factors and early detection and treatment are keys to reducing the debilitating effects of this disease.

Heart Attack and Stroke Prevention

It is important to understand the connection between risk factors and plaque build-up. Risk factors are those things that lead to a clogged artery and include: family history of a heart attack or stroke, male gender, advancing age, abnormal cholesterol, high blood pressure, high blood sugar, smoking, inactivity, excess weight, poor diet, and stress. An irregular heartbeat is also a risk factor for a stroke. Some risk factors can't be changed such as family history and age, but many of the risk factors can be controlled with a healthier lifestyle. A little bit of lifestyle change goes a long way. Your behaviors play a major role in preventing and controlling many of the risk factors that lead to a heart attack or stroke. Each risk factor will be discussed in more detail throughout this book, but first you must understand how a heart attack and stroke develop.

How Blockages Develop

Atherosclerosis is a Latin word that means *athero* (artery) *sclerosis* (hardening.)[1] Plaque is a smaller word that means the same thing. Plaque build-up is a "hardening of the arteries" that can restrict blood flow. I will use the term plaque as I talk about this process and the risk factors that worsen it.

At birth, the inside lining of arteries were smooth, much like the inside of your cheek. Various blood components such as red and white blood cells, platelets, and cholesterol particles traveled through the bloodstream without getting lodged in the lining of the arterial wall. LDL (bad) cholesterol is a type of cholesterol, commonly called bad cholesterol because of its role in heart attack and stroke.

LDL Cholesterol Moving through a Healthy Artery

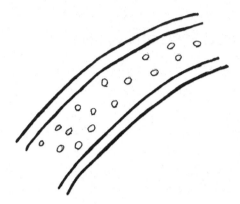

Over time, some wear and tear begins to occur to the inside smooth lining of the artery. Risk factors are those things that cause the damage. In simplest terms, high blood pressure causes a sandpaper effect, making it easier for the LDL (bad) cholesterol to get caught in those roughened areas. High blood sugar scratches the artery walls as it travels through them. Smoking is very toxic because carbon monoxide and other chemicals are carried throughout the arteries. The more damage to the inside lining, the easier it is for the excess LDL (bad) cholesterol to get caught in those damaged areas.

Damaged Arterial Lining

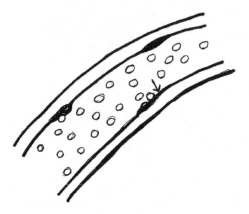

The LDL cholesterol becomes wedged or trapped within the lining wall and does not belong there. The body recognizes this abnormal trapped LDL cholesterol particle as a threat and begins a process to remove it called inflammation. White blood cells go to the damaged area, resulting in an area of redness and inflammation around the trapped LDL particle.

The LDL cholesterol particle is stuck and can't be removed. However, the body keeps trying to remove it and continues to send white blood cells to the area. More and more LDL (bad) cholesterol is caught in the reddened inflamed area along with an army of white blood cells. This process worsens over time. Eventually, calcium deposits form within the plaque as a byproduct of the chronic inflammation.[6] Another term for the calcium build-up is "hardening of the arteries."

Calcium Deposits or Hardening of the Arteries

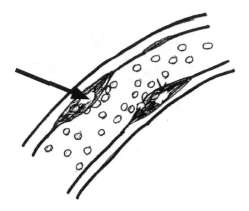

A build-up of plaque causes the artery wall to become weaker and can tear or rupture, causing a heart attack. It is important to remember that a tear can occur with even small amounts of plaque build-up. You do not have to have a large amount of build-up for a heart attack to occur. In fact, most heart attacks occur in people with less than a 50 percent blockage or plaque build-up.[7]

Whenever a blood vessel tears, bleeding follows. The body tries to stop the bleeding by sending sticky particles called platelets to the bleeding area. The platelets stop the bleeding but also clog the artery. Aspirin taken during this time may help reduce the platelets from sticking together. In addition, blood comes in contact with the plaque and a large thrombus, or blood clot, forms. The artery is suddenly completely blocked. No oxygenated blood can get past the blockage. Much like a tourniquet around the arm, pain ensues. If the blockage is not reversed, tissue dies downstream from the obstructed vessel.

Ruptured Wall Causes Blocked Artery or Heart Attack

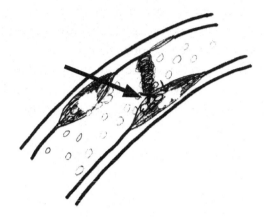

Managing risk factors such as LDL (bad) cholesterol, blood pressure, blood sugar, and not smoking greatly limit the plaque build-up in the arteries. There will be less roughened areas in the arteries and decreased likelihood of LDL getting lodged in the lining. It is never too late to halt the plaque build-up process. Even if you already had a heart attack or stroke, reducing your risk factors will keep the plaque build-up from getting any worse. It is especially important to lower the LDL cholesterol to prevent it from getting caught in damaged areas. When the plaque build-up is halted, a fibrous hardened cap forms over the plaque. This cap protects the underlying weaker artery wall from tearing. By making the artery less likely to tear, risk for a heart attack is reduced. The plaque build-up occurs throughout the body within all of the arteries. In the brain, it leads to strokes; in the kidneys, it causes kidney disease; within the eyes, blindness may ensue; and within the legs, pain with walking. Controlling plaque build-up in one area will reduce the problem throughout the entire body.

Takeaway Points

The good news is that you can halt the plaque progression. But the bad news is that it is much harder to improve disease that has already developed than to prevent it in the first place. In the next chapter, I help you determine your individual risk for a heart attack and stroke and ways to determine if plaque is building up within your arteries. Is your heart a ticking time bomb for an adverse cardiac event?

The oldest and strongest emotion of mankind is fear, and the oldest and strongest kind of fear is fear of the unknown.

—Science Fiction Writer, H. P. Lovecraft

2

Are You at Risk?

Now that you have learned how a heart attack and stroke develop, you may be wondering, "Am I at risk?" In this chapter, I provide you with vital information to calculate your individual risk. While no tool is infallible, it will help you identify the common risk factors for a heart attack and stroke. In general, the greater number of risk factors and their severity, the greater the chance for a cardiac event or stroke. You will also learn about an important screening tool that is available to detect the silent build-up of plaque from a lifetime of harmful behaviors. This chapter ends with surprising stories of famous heart attack and stroke victims. Let's begin this chapter with an overview of the problem and why you should take better care of your arteries.

Overview

Unhealthy eating, a sedentary lifestyle, and frenzied stress have placed Americans at great risk for a heart attack or stroke. While eating out is commonplace, it's important for you to understand the danger. In almost all restaurant food, salt, harmful fat, and sugar are added to make the food taste better. In addition, each entree is large enough to feed three people. Most Americans have grown accustomed to the enhanced taste and keep going back for more. But the salt increases blood pressure while the fat and sugar increase the waistline. The excess weight places a great strain on the heart and body. Inactivity worsens the problem. Most Americans do not have to toil to produce food but spend the vast part of the day sitting behind a desk. You don't even have to get out of your chair to deliver a document to a coworker. You can simply e-mail it. We were not made to sit at a desk all day. Finally, if you are like most people, you are bombarded with an abundance of daily stressors that increase your blood pressure and damage your arteries. Thus, your lifestyle may literally be killing you. It takes years for the arterial plaque build-up to occur. It happens so slowly that you may not be aware of the ticking time bomb building up inside you.

Startling Statistics

Despite the technological advancements in the diagnosis and treatment of heart disease over the past century, it has remained the leading cause of adult deaths.[1] In 2010, approximately, 600,000 people died from heart disease and 130,000 died from a stroke.[1] Roughly speaking, that is equivalent to over four jumbo jets crashing each day, killing all people on board. How do we react when we hear the devastating news of even one airplane crash? Yet we remain in denial about the daily deaths from heart disease.

Interestingly, most women will tell you that they are more concerned about getting breast cancer than having a heart attack or stroke. In reality, the statistics are startling. Only 1 out of 30 women will die from breast cancer while 1 out of 3 will die from heart disease.[1] For men, the statistics are fairly similar as 1 out of 36[2] will die from prostate cancer, but 1 out of 4 will die from heart disease.[3] Are you as diligent about checking your cholesterol levels and blood pressure readings as you are about annual mammograms or prostate exams? In reality, which is the bigger danger?

Further, of those adults who died from sudden cardiac death, 50 percent of men and 64 percent of women had no warning of the impending attack.[1] They were leading normal lives and the first warning sign that there was a problem was a blockage or irregular heart rhythm that completely stopped their heart. In these situations, you have only two or three minutes to get the heart beating again or you die.

New screening technologies exist to identify those at risk for a heart attack, but few take advantage of them. Many people remain in denial, mistakenly believing, "It just won't happen to me." Understandably, the silent nature of atherosclerosis or the plaque build-up process leads many to believe this dangerous conclusion. For others, they may understand that they need to make healthier choices but find the barriers too difficult to overcome. Other people may be unaware of the screening tools available to detect disease.

Denial: The Ostrich

Denying health risks is part of our human nature. We just want to be left alone to live our lives. This attitude is not a new phenomenon. In the 1950s, an outbreak of tuberculosis (TB) occurred. The disease is spread through the air, especially when coughing. Young children, older adults, and chronically ill people are especially vulnerable as their immunity is not as strong to resist the disease. Skin tests were offered throughout the country. If someone's test was positive, a chest X-ray was needed to determine if the person had just been exposed to TB or had an active disease within the lungs. Treatment involved months of various antibiotics. Far too many people avoided the screening test. Despite the war being waged by public health care practitioners to eradicate the disease, it was spreading.

A psychologist, Irwin Rosenstock, wanted to understand why individuals were not participating in tuberculosis screenings and seeking medical treatment if needed. He developed a theory, which is still being used today to understand their denial. His Health Belief Model (HBM) states that the more one thinks that they are at risk for a health problem, the more likely they will take action to do something to reduce their risk.[4]

In this chapter, I hope to increase your knowledge of your risk for a heart attack or stroke. Once you have this information, you can make decisions that will improve your health. Don't be an ostrich and bury your head in the sand. If a problem is identified, there is much that can be done to improve it. Knowledge of your personal risk is the first step so that you will not become a fatal statistic.

Calculate Your Risk

It is important to understand that there are some people who have heart attacks with very few risk factors and others who have many risk factors and never have a heart attack. Truthfully, no one really knows why this happens. Current research is trying to understand this phenomenon. However, most medical evidence, including the landmark Framingham Heart Study, has supported that the greater number of risk factors that you have, the greater your risk for a heart attack or stroke.

Framingham Heart Study

In 1948, physicians noticed an increase in heart attack deaths since the turn of the century. Under the guidance of what is now called the National Heart, Lung, and Blood Institute, scientists in the Framingham Heart Study set out to examine a large population of people. The researchers wanted to determine the risk factors for a heart attack, which were not known at the time. They recruited 5,209 men and women ages 30 to 62 from Framingham, Massachusetts.[5] Every two years, they would be examined, tested, and interviewed. In 1971, the second group of their children and spouses were added to the study, and in 2002, their grandchildren were added. This long-term follow-up has provided invaluable information. Specifically, they wanted to identify the common characteristics of those people who had heart attacks. Those characteristics became known as the risk factors for heart disease. Other studies have supported their findings, and over 1,200 research articles have been written using their data.[5]

When cardiac healthcare providers refer to risk factors for heart disease, they are talking about the characteristics that were revealed from the Framingham study. I will use them to help you calculate your risk. There are two simple methods that can be utilized: Simple Count and the Heart Attack Risk Calculator. No tool is perfect or infallible, but it will help you understand those characteristics that are common in people who have heart disease and whether you have similar traits.

Exception: You Already Had a Heart Attack or Stroke

If you already had a stent placed, heart attack, stroke, or bypass operation, you do not need to complete any of the risk factor calculations because you are automatically at the very highest risk category for a second event. Further, the silent nature of plaque build-up may lead you to some dangerous thinking. A small study examined the thoughts and feelings of women who had a heart attack, angioplasty, or cardiac bypass surgery.[6] The researchers found that the women perceived that once their hearts were "fixed," they no longer had to worry about a heart attack and stroke. The event was so frightening that they just wanted to return to a normal life and not think about it anymore. While their thinking was certainly understandable, plaque build-up is not a static process. It worsens over time unless actions are taken to stop the plaque progression. You must aggressively control all of your risk factors in order to prevent a second event. However, for those of you who have not had a heart attack or stroke, the following methods will help you understand your risk in order to prevent an initial event.

Simple Count Method

The Simple Count Method involves counting your risk factors. The more present, the greater your risk for a heart attack or stroke. I encourage my patients to get a checkup for potential underlying plaque build-up if they have two or more of them.

Check the Risk Factors That Apply to You

Yes	No	Risk Factors
		Genetic Vulnerability Father or brother who had a heart attack or stroke before the age of 55 years or a mother or sister before the age of 65 years.
		Advancing Age You are a male 45 years or older or a female 55 years or older.
		Abnormal Cholesterol Levels Either high amounts of LDL (bad) cholesterol or Low amounts of HDL (good) cholesterol or High amounts of fasting triglycerides over 150.
		High Blood Pressure Pre-high Blood Pressure (120/80-139/89) or High Blood Pressure (over 140/90) or You are taking medications for your blood pressure.
		Elevated Blood Sugar Fasting blood sugar over 100 or non-fasting blood sugar over 140.
		Tobacco Use "Any" amount of cigarettes, cigar, snuff or chewing tobacco.
		Excess Weight Men with a waist measurement over 40 inches or Women with a waist measurement over 35 inches.
		Lack of Physical Activity Aerobic physical activity less than 3 to 4 sessions per week of 30 to 40 minutes of moderate to vigorous intensity (break a sweat).
Total Points_____		The greater number indicates higher risk.

Heart Attack Risk Calculator

The Heart Attack Risk Calculator is the most recent tool.[7] It is based on several variables: gender, age, smoking status, family history of a heart attack or stroke, whether or not you had a heart attack or stroke, evidence of plaque build-up, fasting blood sugar, height, weight, waist measurement, blood pressure, whether or not you are being treated for high blood pressure, total cholesterol, fasting LDL (bad) cholesterol, HDL (good) cholesterol, and fasting triglycerides. The Heart Attack Risk Calculator is an estimate of your potential risk for having a heart attack or stroke within the next ten years.

You may visit https://www.heart.org/gglRisk/main_en_US.html to calculate your risk score. If you score over 7.5 percent, you are considered in the higher risk group and should receive more aggressive screening and treatment. A more extensive explanation of this tool is provided in chapter 3.

The evidence is clear that the more risk factors one has, the greater one's risk for a heart attack and stroke. Either of these tools would be helpful for calculating risk for a heart attack, but they are only estimates. Unfortunately, predicting risk isn't that black and white. Risk factor calculations and stress testing miss many people at risk for a cardiac or stroke event. For patients at high risk, other screening techniques may be more helpful for determining the likelihood of disease.

Problems with Stress Testing Alone

A stress test of any kind involves increasing the heart rate with exercise or medication and watching how the heart responds to the greater workload. The healthcare provider conducting the test looks for any changes in the heart rhythm, blood pressure, and any new symptoms that might develop. During exercise, the body needs more oxygen for the increased activity. If there is a large blockage within a coronary artery, the heart will not be able to keep up with the demands of the extra workload. Usually, the stress test won't reflect a problem unless a blockage within the artery is greater than 70 percent.[8]

Unfortunately, most heart attacks occur in people with blockages less than 50 percent.[8] The stress test would look normal. Patients leave the office feeling good about their results. "I don't have heart disease." A heart attack may still occur because the blood vessels aren't healthy. The test just missed the abnormality.

In my experience, doctors begin with a stress test to ensure that there is not a large blockage greater than 70 percent. Blockages of this severity may need to be opened to prevent more severe problems. If someone with many risk factors or a strong family history has a normal stress test, another test such as the coronary artery calcium heart scan may be done to ensure that something wasn't missed. It is a very accurate measure of how much plaque is building up within the arteries surrounding the outside of the heart.[1]

Coronary Artery Calcium Heart Scan

Doctors have known for a long time about the calcium deposits in the arteries of the heart, but until recently could only see them during an autopsy after someone died, too late to help the patient. Old X-ray and CT scans could not capture clear pictures with a beating heart. In the late 1990s, a new scanning technique was developed to take pictures very rapidly in between heartbeats when the heart was briefly at rest. The calcium deposits or hardening of the arteries could be seen clearly and measured. At a glance, the doctor could determine how much plaque was present based on the amount of calcium deposits visible on the scan.[9] If a patient has a great deal of calcium deposits, their body is vulnerable for either a heart attack or stroke. The coronary artery calcium heart scan (CAC) is a marker for a gross measurement of plaque accumulation in the arteries.[1] It is important to understand the association of coronary calcium deposits as they are related to plaque build-up.

Coronary Calcium and Plaque Build-Up

Plaque build-up or atherosclerosis often begins in childhood and progresses with age. Recall that the LDL (bad) cholesterol is the main target of therapy because LDL becomes trapped within the inside lining of the arteries. As already described in chapter 1, the body fights a war (inflammation) to remove the trapped LDL cholesterol particle. However, it cannot be removed. Eventually, calcium deposits form during this process of inflammation.

The plaque that is present is in various stages of the build up process and the calcium deposits represent the older plaque. The arteries surrounding the heart should not have any calcium deposits. Because calcium is the main component of bone, these deposits look like bone. The calcified plaques that are visualized with this technology represent about 20 percent of the overall plaque.[9] The results do not show where a potential blockage may be located, only how much overall disease is present. If you are someone with a great amount of plaque, you are also someone at much greater risk for a heart attack or stroke. This information is powerful and has the potential to save many lives. The non-contrast scan is a quick noninvasive test that takes a few minutes to complete and has the equivalent dose of radiation as a mammogram.[10]

Calcium Deposits in the Coronary Arteries (Santos)[11]

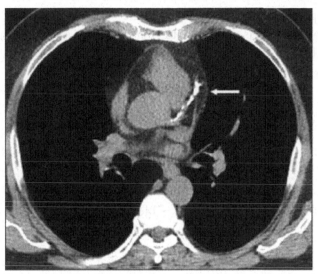

Fig. 1 - Calcification of the anterior descending artery detected on ultrafast tomography in an asymptomatic man (arrow).

Who Should Get a Scan

The test is not recommended for persons who already had an angioplasty with a stent placed, a heart bypass operation or had a heart attack, as you are already in the highest risk category. Currently, a coronary artery calcium heart scan is recommended for adults who are found to be at intermediate risk.[12] This practice is endorsed by the American Heart Association, and the American College of Cardiology. The most recent 2013 Guidelines of the Assessment of Cardiovascular Risk state that the test may help clarify risk.[13] Despite this support and endorsement, the test is still underutilized, which is why I am covering it in such detail in this book. It is available in most major cities and I think that any male over forty-five years old or female over fifty-five years should get a baseline test. The cost of the non-contrast coronary artery calcium heart scan is around $400.[14] However, costs have been coming down, approaching $100 in some centers. Most facilities offer special discounts throughout the year, but especially during February, which is dedicated to the awareness and eradication of heart disease. Ask for a discounted rate when you call to schedule your test.

How Often Should I Get a Coronary Artery Calcium Heart Scan?

According to noted prevention cardiologist and author of the *South Beach Diet* books, Dr. Arthur Agatston describes his recommendations for the test. He also developed the scoring system used to interpret the results.[15]

> I've found that a compelling visual provides strong motivation for patients to stay on their treatment program, and in particular to keep taking their medications. Moreover, follow-up heart scans can help you and your doctor keep track of your progress and make the necessary adjustments to your treatment program if need be. If you have few or no calcium deposits, you need not repeat the heart scan for at least 5 years. If you do have signs of calcium buildup, the test can be repeated every 2 to 5 years, depending on your other risk factors. (217)

The research is still emerging regarding how far apart the tests should be done. Your healthcare provider who knows you best may have a different view of how frequent you should or should not be rechecked. Getting blood tests and blood pressure checks to ensure that your risk factors are under control is vital. While there are no absolutes, if you are aggressively controlling your risk factors, you are most likely keeping the plaque build-up in check as well.

Radiation Exposure

A word of caution is needed. The screening calcium test is the equivalent of a mammogram and the information provided readily identifies patients that require aggressive lifestyle and medication modification. However, intravenous (IV) contrast dye can image the non-calcified plaque as well. The images are almost as clear as an angiogram, as the contrast flows through the arteries and is much less invasive. However, it takes a great deal of radiation, equal to 600 chest X-rays, to get those pictures.[16] My recommendation is to stick with the simple non-contrast coronary artery calcium heart scan every few years or so to ensure that the plaque build-up has slowed and avoid the CT angiogram. Of course, your healthcare provider may have sound reasons for the more extensive test. Do your homework and ask a lot of questions of your healthcare provider. You are the consumer. Good clinicians will appreciate your interest and concern.

A Word about an Inflammation Blood Test

Some healthcare providers use a test to measure the inflammation caused from the plaque build-up. When inflammation occurs in the body, chemicals are released and can be measured in the blood. High Sensitivity C Reactive Protein (hs-CRP) is a simple blood test that can measure the amount of one such inflammation marker. It is said that there is a correlation between the amount found in the blood and the level of inflammation. Proponents argue that hs-CRP is a quick and inexpensive way to determine plaque build-up. In some practices, it is being used to monitor change after starting medication or lifestyle treatment. Opponents counter that labs do not uniformly measure the test and results vary. The biggest criticisms have been that the test can't distinguish the cause of the inflammation. Is it heart disease, arthritis, or a toothache? In theory, it would be very helpful to find a simple blood test that identifies plaque build-up; however, their clinical usefulness is still being investigated. Research is ongoing to identify better predictors of those at risk for a heart attack or stroke.

Celebrities Who Died Too Young

There are many celebrities who have experienced a heart attack or stroke. Some died suddenly, but their deaths could have been prevented with better lifestyle choices. Others received a huge wake-up call to make changes. These stories are only a few of the millions of Americans who suffer from heart disease.

James Fixx

Fixx was an avid marathon runner who died from a massive heart attack at age fifty-two in 1984.[17] He wrote a book titled *The Complete Book of Running* and was credited with initiating the running craze. He ran ten miles a day and played an aggressive game of tennis the day before he died. His death sent shock waves throughout the runner and medical community. What happened?

Before he started running, he spent years as a heavy man who smoked two packs of cigarettes a day.[17] He quit seventeen years before his death. Any type of tobacco use causes severe damage to the arteries throughout the body. He also had a very strong family history of premature heart disease. His father's first attack occurred at age thirty-five and he died at forty-three years old. Fixx did not have a relationship with a doctor and didn't seek medical care. His autopsy showed a massive amount of plaque build-up. Early detection and medical treatment probably would have saved his life. His wife stated, "He never had any warning." When writing about the death of James Fixx, Dr. Lawrence Altman wrote:

But the insidious thing about heart disease, which is the nation's leading cause of death, is that it is often so secret and veiled that doctors cannot always detect severe cases such as Mr. Fixx's from routine tests.[17] (1)

James Gandolfini

Gandolfini known for his role in *The Sopranos* was overweight, smoked cigars, was a binge eater, and had a great deal of stress.[18] While vacationing in Italy, he ate a large meal of shrimp and foie gras, very high in harmful fats and salt, which probably caused undo stress on his heart. The strain of digesting this meal appeared to push him into cardiac arrest in front of his terrified thirteen-year-old son. He died at fifty-one years old.

Near Misses

David Letterman

Letterman, the host of *Late Night with David Letterman*, jogged six miles the day before he had his bypass operation.[19] He smoked cigars and had a very strong family history of premature heart disease as well. He joked that his "total cholesterol was borderline at 680." The actual number was not reported. A stress test indicated an abnormality, which led to an angiogram and a subsequent quintuple (five) bypass operation in 2000 at age fifty-two.

George W. Bush

While in office, President Bush was known to push his secret service agents to keep up with him in vigorous exercise. He was under the care and supervision of excellent doctors and was in great shape. A routine stress test indicated an abnormality, and though he did not have any symptoms, an angiogram was ordered. This test indicated a 95 percent blockage.[20] Despite his phenomenal physical activity, he had an angioplasty with a stent placement to prevent him from a future catastrophic cardiac event.

A Word about Stroke

Dick Clark

Clark was known as "the world's oldest teenager" because of his youthful appearance. He had a history of heart disease and type 2 diabetes.[21] He suffered a stroke in 2004 from plaque build-up in his brain. It resulted in a severe speech impediment, and he died in 2012 from a massive heart attack. A stroke is a devastating disease, which impacts quality of life profoundly. There are many types of impairment. It just depends on the location of the damaged artery.

Sharon Stone

Recall that Dick Clark's type of stroke was caused by a clotting problem and is the most common. However, it is also good to learn what happened to Sharon Stone who had a bleeding stroke in 2001 at age forty-three.[22] An artery ruptured and she almost died. While these types of strokes are less common, high blood pressure can greatly increase their occurrence. Stone was in great physical shape, training for a three-mile charity run. She noticed a crippling headache that brought her to the doctor. A CT scan of her brain located the bleeding artery, which was repaired. She suffered a severe speech impediment and stated that "I lost the feeling of my left leg to my knee for 8 months."[23] She worked hard in rehabilitation to get her function back. These stories represent the impact from a heart attack and stroke, but many Americans remain at risk as well. Denial of the potential danger is a major problem.

Farmer Story

One of my former patients illustrates the importance of screening and working with a healthcare provider. He had an extremely high amount of plaque build-up that was detected with a coronary artery calcium heart scan. I reviewed his results while his wife was present. She stated, "Nurse, your information is very helpful, but I don't think that my husband will follow up with his doctor. He thinks that every time he goes to the doctor, they always find something wrong. The last time he went to a doctor was 20 years ago. He doesn't think that he has a problem now."

This was a classic example of denial. So I asked the farmer, "What would happen if you left your tractor out in the field for a year, for 5 years, for 20 years (the last time he saw a doctor), and you did nothing to maintain the tractor?"

He said, "Well the tractor would be a mess."

I replied, "Your body is just like your tractor. Maintenance is important. If a problem is caught early, there is much that can be done. But if you leave it alone for 20 years, you could be in a lot of trouble." Eventually, the patient moved out of his denial, followed up with his doctor and began treatment to prevent an event. It was a close call for him as he was very close to having a heart attack.

Don't be like the farmer with your head in the sand. For many patients, their first warning was sudden death. I recommend that if you are a male over forty-five years old or a female over fifty-five years old, you should talk with your healthcare provider about obtaining a baseline cardiac screening. I favor the non-contrast coronary artery calcium heart scan because of the low cost, low risk, and reliability. It just may save your life. If you are experiencing any of the symptoms for a heart attack or stroke discussed in chapter 1, call 911. Be safe rather than sorry and don't be like the celebrities and farmer in the previous stories.

Takeaway Points

Medical research continues to move forward, and each year, more is learned about predicting those who are at increased risk. In this chapter, I covered the most accurate tools that are supported by the recent guidelines. Many more are emerging. If you have questions about other tests that were not covered within this chapter or need help in locating a coronary artery calcium heart scan close to you, please feel free to contact me through my Web site (www.living4ahealthyheart.com). Hopefully, you now understand the cause of a heart attack or stroke and the significant role that risk factors play in their development. Armed with this information, you can apply it to your daily life with the goal of preventing heart disease. There is no better time than now to find out if you are in danger of a heart attack or stroke and get your risk factors under control!

An apple a day keeps the doctor away.

—Pembrokeshire Proverb

3

Cholesterol: The Good, the Bad, End the Confusion

Understanding the Numbers

Heart disease remains the number 1 killer of adults in America, with abnormal cholesterol playing a major role.[1] At the turn of the last century, the average life expectancy was forty-seven years old.[2] A variety of medications and treatments have changed the life expectancy in 2011 to seventy-six years for men and eighty-one years for women.[2] Much of that increased lifespan can be attributed to the development of antibiotics and cholesterol-lowering drugs.

Lifestyle is also extremely important. The healthier life you live, the less medication you will need. However, quality of life is also important. Each person must decide what behaviors that they are willing to change in order to decrease their risk for a heart attack or stroke. For many people, it may be too hard to eat a perfectly healthy diet all of the time. For others, the genetic factors are so abnormal that no amount of lifestyle sacrifices are enough to keep the risk low. For all of these patients, medications can be given to lower the risk. Medications can be very effective, but they may come with annoying side effects. Ultimately, the decision rests with you and what you are willing to do to reduce your risk—healthier lifestyle, medication, or both. I begin this chapter with an overview of cholesterol and an explanation of what the different numbers mean.

Cholesterol

Cholesterol is a fatty molecule that is present in the body and bloodstream. It is carried through the blood on fat molecules called lipoproteins. The body needs a small amount of cholesterol for hormone production, cell formation, and digestion. The amount of cholesterol in the bloodstream is primarily based upon the amount made by the liver. The liver's production of cholesterol is mainly determined by genetics and, to a smaller degree, the food that you eat. Saturated fats, which are solid at room temperature, may raise blood cholesterol levels.

What Do the Numbers Mean?

There are several lab values that are measured on a fasting lipid profile or cholesterol blood test: total cholesterol, HDL (good) cholesterol, LDL (bad) cholesterol, VLDL (very bad) cholesterol and triglycerides. A blood sugar test is often measured at the same time. I recommend that you get your most recent blood test results and compare them to the information that I provide throughout this section. It was adapted from the National Cholesterol Education Program, Adult Treatment Panel III Guidelines,[3] and the 2005 updates.[4]

Values of a Lipid Profile (Cholesterol Test)

Total Cholesterol (Keep Lower)	
Less than 200	Desirable
200-239	Borderline high
Greater than or equal to 240	High
LDL (Bad) Cholesterol (Keep Lower)	
Less than 100	Optimal
100-129	Near optimal/above optimal
130-159	Borderline high
160-189	High
Above or equal to 190	Very high
Less than 70	Optimal for very high risk patients
HDL (Good) Cholesterol (Keep Higher)	
Less than 40	High Risk
Above or equal to 60	Optimal
Triglycerides (Keep Lower)	
Less than 150	Normal
150-199	Borderline high
200-499	High
Above or equal to 500	Very high

*High risk patients had a heart attack, stroke, have diabetes, have been told that plaque is building-up or have several risk factors.
*National Cholesterol Education Panel (NCEP, ATP III)

LDL (Bad) Cholesterol

The LDL or low density lipoproteins are "bad" because they may become trapped within the walls of the arteries and cause plaque build-up. Thus, the LDL (bad) cholesterol is the most important number for you to remember and monitor over time.

VLDL (Very Bad) Cholesterol

While the VLDL value is often not listed within a cholesterol test, I did want to provide you with some information on it. The VLDL or very low density lipoproteins are included within the total cholesterol number but rarely mentioned. It gets the name "very bad" as it easily becomes lodged within the arterial wall and is worse than LDL (bad) cholesterol. The VLDL number fluctuates and is more difficult to use in clinical practice, which is why it is generally not discussed.

HDL (Good) Cholesterol

The HDL or high density lipoproteins are labeled "good" because they scoop up the bad cholesterol and carry it back to the liver where the body can get rid of it. I think of HDL (good) cholesterol as the garbage men and the LDL (bad) cholesterol and VLDL (very bad) cholesterol as the garbage. If you do not have enough garbage collectors, you need to reduce the amount of garbage to prevent garbage build-up. Exercise increases HDL (good) cholesterol while smoking lowers it. Genetics plays a very big role as well. In some people, their livers do not make enough HDL (good) cholesterol despite healthy lifestyle choices.

It is also important to remember that if you are someone with high levels of HDL (good) cholesterol but your LDL cholesterol levels remain high, something may be going on that causes you to still have too much LDL (bad) cholesterol circulating in your blood. This situation is still not completely understood. It is important to remember that keeping your LDL (bad) cholesterol number under control is still the goal no matter how much HDL (good) cholesterol you have.[3] You may have a high amount of good guys, but the bad guys are winning the war. For these people, medications may be needed to lower the bad cholesterol.

Total Cholesterol

The total cholesterol is made up of all three: LDL (bad), VLDL (very bad), and HDL (good). The total cholesterol value is not very helpful because it represents a mix of all three. Therefore, I think it is more important to know how much bad cholesterol you have compared to the good levels.

Triglycerides

Although triglycerides are not included in the total cholesterol number, they are generally reported as part of the blood work. Triglycerides are used to calculate the LDL (bad) cholesterol number. I think of triglycerides as a type of liquid fat that moves through the blood. If you eat a diet high in cookies, ice cream, and alcohol, your body converts those foods to liquid fat. You have about twenty-four hours to burn it for fuel or they are converted to stored fat. It's important to note that you must fast for at least twelve hours prior to measuring your triglycerides in order to get an accurate level.

High triglycerides, low HDL (good) cholesterol, and excess belly fat are often seen before diabetes is diagnosed.[4] Refer to chapter 5 for a longer discussion on diabetes and pre-diabetes. I tell patients that this is a red flag warning that diabetes is imminent if they don't make changes to correct these abnormal numbers. Reducing sweets and alcohol and increasing physical activity helps to burn excess fat for fuel. I provide tips regarding sugar and alcohol in chapter 6 when I talk about weight management.

Medications also help lower triglycerides. Very high triglycerides (over 500) may indicate a serious inflammation or swelling of the pancreas and requires medical attention immediately![3]

Knowing your numbers and what they mean is the first step in controlling your cholesterol and reducing your risk for a heart attack and stroke, but unfortunately, it is not enough. Until recently, healthcare providers believed that if the LDL (bad) cholesterol was lowered to less than 100 or less than 70 for high risk patients, heart attack, and stroke risk was profoundly decreased. Recent studies have shown that for some people, those numbers are not low enough. The most recent guidelines reflect this new research.[5] The following example of one study will help you understand why the guidelines were adjusted.

Puzzling Findings

A very large national study examined the medical records (541 hospitals) of 136,905 patients hospitalized with a heart attack between 2000 and 2006 who had a cholesterol test done on admission.[6] The researchers were surprised to find that the patients had fairly low LDL (bad) cholesterol numbers. Half of the heart attack patients had an LDL (bad) cholesterol level below 100, while 18 percent were below 70. Only 21 percent were taking cholesterol lowering medications to get those numbers down. Why would people with lower LDL (bad) cholesterol levels have heart attacks? What do these findings suggest? It may be that the LDL (bad) cholesterol goal needs to be lower than 100 since they had heart attacks with low numbers. Researchers are also looking into the size of the LDL particle as smaller ones become lodged more easily. The size of the LDL was not measured in this study. Interestingly, half of the patients had HDL (good) cholesterol levels that were too low, below 40. Only 10 percent had HDL (good) cholesterol numbers above 60. The scientists wondered if low levels of HDL (good) cholesterol play a more vital role in heart attack risk than previously thought.

LDL (bad) cholesterol trapped in the arterial wall is the problem, but some people with low levels have heart attacks while others with higher LDL levels do not. It has remained a mystery. An expert panel of cholesterol specialists examined current research on cholesterol to determine why this can occur. You may find a copy of the 2013 American College of Cardiology (ACC)/American Heart Association (AHA) Guideline on the Treatment of Blood Cholesterol by visiting www.americanheart. org or www.nhlbi.gov.

The experts found that the people taking high doses of cholesterol lowering medications such as statins had fewer heart attacks and strokes. It didn't matter what the LDL value was before treatment. The important factor was to drop LDL (bad) cholesterol by 50 percent in high risk individuals.[5] In the face of these findings, the expert team changed the entire guidelines. Recall in chapter 1 how the LDL (bad) cholesterol travels through the blood and becomes lodged in the arterial wall. Lowering LDL cholesterol helps prevent further build-up and damage.

Healthy Eating to Improve Blood Cholesterol Levels

The 2013 cholesterol guidelines[5] still recommend a healthy lifestyle: heart healthy eating, regular exercise, avoidance of tobacco products, and maintaining a healthy weight. Diabetes, exercise, tobacco cessation, and weight are discussed in upcoming chapters.

While you may have inherited a body that makes too much LDL (bad) cholesterol or triglycerides, dietary factors can worsen an underlying problem. There are three types of fats that impact your blood cholesterol numbers: saturated fat, polyunsaturated fats, and monounsaturated fats.[3] Saturated fats are harmful because they raise LDL (bad) cholesterol. Polyunsaturated fats (oils) are recommended but may lower the HDL (good) cholesterol. Monounsaturated fats are the fats of choice, as they do not increase LDL (bad) cholesterol or lower HDL (good) cholesterol. I spend most of the following section discussing saturated fats since they are the most problematic at increasing your LDL.

Saturated Fat

Saturated fats generally come from animals and are solid at room temperature: butter, lard, marbling on meats, milk, and dairy fat. Coconut and palm oils are also saturated fats. After eating a saturated fat, it becomes LDL (bad) cholesterol in the bloodstream and therefore should be avoided as much as possible.

Amount of Saturated Fat Grams in Foods[7]

Food	Saturated Fat Grams (g)
Dairy Products	
Butter (1 Tablespoon)	7
Margarine (1 T)	1
Whole milk (1 cup)	5
Skim milk (1 cup)	0.3
Plain low fat yogurt (1 cup)	2.3
Cheddar cheese (1 ounce)	6
Meats	
Salmon baked (3 oz.)	1.6
Halibut baked (3 oz.)	0.4
Skinless chicken breast baked (without skin) (3 oz.)	1.2
Beef short ribs (3 oz.)	17
Hotdog (standard)	7
Junk Food	
French Fries (small order)	4
Cheese cake (small piece)	9
Step by Step: Eating To Lower Your Blood Cholesterol U.S. Department of Health and Human Services	

According to the 2013 cholesterol guidelines, less than 5 to 6 percent of your fat intake should consist of saturated fats.[5] I think that it is too complex to try and calculate this number. It might be easier to pay attention to saturated fat "grams." The recommended saturated fat gram intake varies depending on the amount of calories that you consume per day. If you take in 2,000 calories a day, you should limit your saturated fat gram intake to less than 16 grams a day.[8] It is easy to eat too much in one day. Visit the American Heart Association Web site for their specific diet recommendations at www.americanheart.org.

In my experience, most patients find a less than 6 percent saturated fat diet just too hard to follow. They might start with the best intentions, but this diet becomes difficult and they feel a tremendous amount of guilt when they fail to remain on it. One more failure. Simply start by looking at the food label and making very small changes so that you will be successful. Every little bit helps!

Simple Food Label Strategies

Reading food labels can become overly complicated, but I do think it can be helpful if you keep it simple. The following example illustrates helpful information found on a label. As you look at the following labels, just pay attention to those lines that are highlighted. For now, everything else is really not needed.

Brand A and Brand B Saturated Fat Food Label

Chocolate Ice Cream Brand A		Chocolate Ice Cream Brand B	
Serving Size	½ cup	Serving Size	½ cup
Calories per serving	260	Calories per serving	100
Total fat	17(g)	Total fat	3.5(g)
Saturated fat	10(g)	Saturated fat	2(g)
Trans fat	0.5(g)	Trans fat	0(g)
Cholesterol	90(mg)	Cholesterol	15(mg)
Sodium	45(mg)	Sodium	30(mg)
Total carbohydrates	22(g)	Total carbohydrates	15(g)
Dietary fiber	0(g)	Dietary fiber	1(g)
Sugars	19(g)	Sugars	13(g)
Protein	5(g)	Protein	3(g)

First, look at the serving size. The label contains the food information for each serving size. In this example, 1 serving = 1/2 cup. This piece of information is very important and commonly misleading. If you ate 1 cup of ice cream, you would need to double the calories, etc. In the past, food manufacturers would list an unreasonable serving size, such as ½ of a candy bar, when in reality, most people would consume the entire amount. Always pay attention to the amount of food you eat when compared to the listed serving size. Evaluating the saturated fat content is very important, as your body will convert this fat to cholesterol. Brand B is the healthier option since it contains less saturated fat grams. Initially, the lower fat content may not taste as delectable; however, over time, your taste buds will adjust. You can satisfy the ice cream fix without the added saturated fat and calories.

Milk Example

My husband loved whole milk when we got married. I encouraged him to switch to skim milk. The saturated fat content in one cup of whole milk is 5 grams, while it is 0 grams for skim milk. At first, he didn't like the flavor, but over time, he learned to love skim milk.

Milk Food Labels

Whole Milk		2 % Milk		Skim Milk	
Serving size	1 cup	Serving size	1 cup	Serving size	1 cup
Calories per serving	160	Calories per serving	140	Calories per serving	90
Total fat	8 (g)	Total fat	5(g)	Total fat	0(g)
Saturated fat	5(g)	Saturated fat	3(g)	Saturated fat	0(g)
Trans fat	0(g)	Trans fat	0(g)	Trans fat	0(g)
Cholesterol	35(mg)	Cholesterol	25(mg)	Cholesterol	3(mg)
Sodium	125(mg)	Sodium	150(mg)	Sodium	130(mg)
Total carbohydrates	13(g)	Total carbohydrates	15(g)	Total carbohydrates	13(g)
Dietary fiber	0(g)	Dietary fiber	0(g)	Dietary fiber	0(g)
Sugars	12(g)	Sugars	14(g)	Sugars	12(g)
Protein	8(g)	Protein	10(g)	Protein	9(g)

You can see that the saturated fat content is much greater in the whole milk compared to the 2 percent and skim milk. If you are interested in weaning off whole milk, try mixing half whole milk with half 2 percent milk for a while, then switch to 2 percent milk. After a few weeks, mix the 2 percent milk with the skim milk for a while; after some time, switch to skim milk. Go slowly as you will adjust to the taste of milk with less saturated fat.

Trans-Fats (Butter Versus Margarine)

You may be confused about whether you should use butter or margarine. The research seems to go back and forth. At first, scientists thought that since the saturated fat in butter was bad, margarine would be better. Later, scientists found that the trans-fats in the margarine were an even larger problem. Trans-fats are added to margarine to keep it from spoiling and are not found naturally. People became confused. The bottom line for you is to read the labels and try the spread that has the lowest amount of saturated fat that your taste will allow and the least amount of trans-fats. The American Heart Association recommends that a person on a 2,000 calorie diet eat less than 2 grams of trans-fats a day.[9] I instruct my patients to eat as little as possible. As you examine the following food label, pay attention to the highlighted areas.

Butter, Margarine, and Light Butter with Canola Oil Food Label

Butter		Margarine		Light Butter with Canola Oil	
Serving size	1 Tab.	Serving size	1 Tab.	Serving size	1 Tab.
Calories per serving	100	Calories per serving	100	Calories per serving	50
Total Fat	11(g)	Total fat	11(g)	Total fat	5(g)
Saturated fat	7(g)	Saturated fat	2(g)	Saturated fat	2(g)
Trans fat	0(g)	Trans fat	2.5(g)	Trans fat	0(g)
Cholesterol	30(mg)	Cholesterol	0(mg)	Cholesterol	5(mg)
Sodium	90(mg)	Sodium	105(mg)	Sodium	90(mg)
Total carbohydrates	0(g)	Total carbohydrates	0(g)	Total carbohydrates	0(g)
Dietary fiber	0(g)	Dietary fiber	0(g)	Dietary fiber	0(g)
Sugars	0(g)	Sugars	0(g)	Sugars	0(g)
Protein	0(g)	Protein	0(g)	Protein	0(g)

First look at what is considered a serving: 1 Tablespoon or 1 pat of butter. How much butter do you use when you apply it to your toast? Do you typically use only 1 pat? Butter has 7 grams of saturated fat, high in saturated fats, but no trans-fats. Margarine contains 2 grams of saturated fat, which is better, but it also has 2.5 grams of trans-fats. The light butter made with canola oil has only 2 grams of saturated fat with no trans-fats, which is the best choice. These products are becoming more popular because they are better for your heart.

The Red Velvet Cake Story

My husband's coworker made a red velvet cake that everyone at the office raved about. He was very proud of this cake and made it for many of the lunch events. I made his red velvet cake to understand why it was so good. It had six sticks of real butter in it. I calculated that each single serving probably had between 18 and 23 grams of saturated fat, not to mention 2 ounces of artificial red food coloring added to the cake. One piece of cake had more than an entire day's allowance of saturated fat but tasted like a luxurious dessert from a very expensive restaurant. I learned firsthand that the extraordinary flavor came from all that butter.

I've spent a great deal of time reviewing saturated fats, as they are the worst food offender for increasing your LDL (bad) cholesterol. It is most likely ending up in your blood, increasing your risk for a heart attack and stroke. Awareness is the first step. My simple strategy of focusing on the saturated fat portion of the label will help you improve your diet choices without changing your quality of life. Have fun with reading labels as you experiment with different types of lower saturated fat foods. Make simple reductions and see how your LDL (bad) cholesterol responds. You can experiment with making healthier versions by substituting high calorie ingredients for lower calorie ones. Eat rich desserts sparingly, and if you have a poor diet day, try to eat healthier the next day. Remember, your goal may be to try the food item that is healthier. You can still enjoy the taste without all of the harm to your arteries.

Polyunsaturated Fat (Oils)

Polyunsaturated fats are vegetable oils such as safflower oil, sunflower, soybean, or corn oil. The polyunsaturated oils that occur naturally in fish such as salmon are especially good for you. The American Heart Association (AHA) recommends that you eat fish at least two times a week. However, be sure that you avoid fish contaminated with mercury.[10] You can visit www.americanheart.org for a list of fish that may be high in mercury and should be avoided. The AHA also provides a list of the fish that are safe to eat and good for you.

Monounsaturated Fat (Oils)

Monounsaturated fats such as canola oil and olive oil are the best to use. I use canola oil for baking and olive oil for salad dressings and stir-frys. When eating out at a restaurant, a good idea is to dip your bread in olive oil and grated parmesan cheese instead of butter.

Living for a Healthy Heart Plan

My philosophy is to keep it simple. The following is the Living for a Healthy Heart Plan, which is a summary of many of the healthy diet recommendations. This diet is higher in fruits and vegetables and helps to prevent a heart attack, stroke, cancer, and many other chronic diseases that result from poor eating. Start with any of the following healthier options whenever you can.

Living for A Healthy Heart Plan

- **Eat**
  - a plant-based diet of more fruits and vegetables.
  - whole grains, beans and dark rice.
  - lean meats the size of a deck of cards no more than twice a day.
  - lower fat dairy products such as skim milk.
  - olive or canola oil.
  - palm size of nuts a day for one snack.

- **Reduce**
  - processed foods and saturated fats in your diet.
  - desserts and sugary drinks.
  - salt.
  - alcohol.
  - portion sizes.

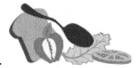

- **Hydrate**
  - by drinking more water.

Remember to be realistic, start small, and go slow. Don't try to change your entire diet at once. It may be too much. Be realistic about what you can change. Food is important to your quality of life. I love chocolate, but I also know that it is high in saturated fat and calories. I eat a palm-size of chocolate-covered almonds or chocolate-covered dried fruit. The key is the palm size! I am able to satisfy my chocolate craving and still take care of my heart. I also love cheddar cheese. I buy the strongest flavor of extra sharp cheddar cheese and cut a thin slice of it. The stronger flavor still gives me the taste of the cheddar cheese with a smaller amount of saturated fat. The important concept to understand here is to think about what you are able to change and start very slow and small. Remember, all changes help. Your job is to decide just how much you are able to do with your diet. The rest will have to be adjusted with medication. The choice remains with you.

Medications: When Diet Isn't Enough

A healthier diet remains very important in controlling cholesterol numbers in order to reduce risk for a heart attack or stroke. However, sometimes, it isn't enough and medications are required. While the 2013 cholesterol guidelines emphasize the importance of a healthier lifestyle, the experts placed a much higher emphasis on profoundly decreasing LDL (bad) cholesterol with medications. These guidelines were endorsed by several prominent organizations: American Heart Association, American College of Cardiology, American Association of Cardiovascular and Pulmonary Rehabilitation, American Pharmacists, American Society of Preventive Cardiologists, Association of Black Cardiologists, Preventive Cardiovascular Nurses Association and WomenHeart: The National Coalition for Women with Heart Disease.

2013 Cholesterol Guidelines for Medication Treatment[5]

The 2013 cholesterol guidelines call for more aggressive lowering of LDL (bad) cholesterol among four groups of people: those with a prior history of a heart attack or stroke, those with LDL (bad) cholesterol over 190, persons with diabetes and LDL levels over 70, and high risk people without a previous heart attack or stroke history. People that fall into one of these four groups are at greater risk. The treatment goals are designed to lower LDL values regardless of the baseline LDL. Aggressive treatment involves high dose statin therapy. Statin medications block an enzyme that is needed for the liver to make cholesterol.[11] "High-intensity statin treatment" lowers LDL more than 50 percent, "moderate-intensity statin treatment" lowers LDL between 30 percent to 50 percent, and "low-intensity statin treatment" lowers LDL less than 30 percent.[5]

Statin Treatment[5]

High-Intensity	Moderate-Intensity	Low-Intensity
Lowers LDL 50% or more	Lowers LDL 30% to <50%	Lowers LDL <30%
Atorvastatin 40-80 mg Rosuvastatin 20-40 mg	Atorvastatin 10-20 mg Rosuvastatin 5-10 mg Simvastatin 20-40 mg Pravastatin 40-80 mg Lovastatin 40 mg Fluvastatin XL 80 mg Fluvastatin 40 mg bid Pitavastatin 2-4 mg	Simvastatin 10 mg Pravastatin 10-20 mg Lovastatin 20 mg Fluvastatin 20-40 mg Pitavastatin 1 mg

While a healthy lifestyle is important, medical therapy is the first step for people that are in one of the four groups.

Four Highest Risk Groups

1. Prior History of a Heart Attack or Stroke

The people most likely to suffer a second heart attack or stroke are those people that have already had one. High-intensity statin treatment and healthier lifestyle changes will reduce risk for another event. In general, whatever the LDL value was at the time of your event, it needs to be decreased by 50 percent afterward.[5] This recommendation applies if you have a history of an abdominal aortic aneurysm, peripheral arterial disease (plaque build-up) in your legs, a high coronary artery calcium heart scan score (over 300), angioplasty with stent placement or you had a heart bypass operation.

2. LDL (Bad) Cholesterol over 190

Some people are born with livers that produce dangerously high amounts of LDL (bad) cholesterol. Because the liver works in overdrive, dietary changes are not enough to slow the formation of excess LDL, making medication necessary.

3. Persons with Diabetes with LDL Levels over 70

Excess blood sugar scratches the arterial walls as it travels through the blood. It is easier for the LDL cholesterol to become trapped and cause plaque build-up. If you have diabetes with many risk factors, you should have high-intensity statin treatment that drops your LDL number by half.[5] If you have diabetes with only a few risk factors, you should receive "moderate intensity statin treatment" to decrease your LDL by a third. [5] Your healthcare provider will determine your risk and appropriate treatment, based on your number of risk factors.

4. High Risk People without a Previous Heart Attack or Stroke History

Some people have so many risk factors and a strong family history that they are at great risk. If treated early with medications and lifestyle changes, a heart attack and stroke may be prevented. The 2013 guideline experts developed a tool to identify those with enough risk factors to require high-intensity statin treatment.

Heart Attack Risk Calculator[5]

The Heart Attack Risk Calculator is an estimate of your potential risk for having a heart attack or stroke within the next ten years. It is not an absolute measurement but rather compares you with other people your age and gender. Remember that your healthcare provider remains the very best person to discuss your individual situation and determine your risk.

You may visit https://www.heart.org/gglRisk/main_en_US.html to calculate your risk score. You will be asked to supply the following information: gender, age, smoking status, family history of heart attack and stroke, whether or not you personally experienced a heart attack, stroke, or have diabetes, blood sugar over 100, height, weight, waist measurement over 35 inches for women, and over 40 inches for men, blood pressure, whether or not you are being treated for high blood pressure, total cholesterol, LDL (bad) cholesterol, HDL (good) cholesterol, and whether your triglycerides are over 150. You are given a percentage number that indicates the likelihood of you having a heart attack or stroke within the next ten years. If you score over 7.5 percent, you are considered in a high risk group and should receive high-intensity statin treatment along with lifestyle changes to protect you. If you have a score less than 7.5 percent, your healthcare provider will examine your risk factors for appropriate treatment, but lifestyle changes remain very important.

The Importance of Statins

The guideline experts examined the research to date and found that those patients who took statins had significantly less heart attack and strokes compared to those who did not take this medication. Statins are the most effective medication to profoundly lower LDL (bad) cholesterol.[5] Because the action is in the liver, regular blood tests are needed to monitor the liver for any potential problems. The Food and Drug Administration (FDA) issued a warning for healthcare providers to use caution when prescribing a high dose of 80 mgs of Simvastatin (Zocor) to patients.[12] High doses may disrupt the liver leading to a rare muscle breakdown disorder called rhabdomyolysis. The FDA advises patients to contact their healthcare provider immediately if they notice "muscle pain, tenderness or weakness, dark or red-colored urine, or unexpected fatigue." Blood tests can be done to check for the disorder and abnormal liver function. Kidney damage is also a dangerous complication.

However, the FDA does not want people to stop taking their statins because of this warning. Dr. Eric Coleman, the deputy director of the FDA's Division of Metabolism and Endocrinology Products, states, "The benefits of the treatment far outweigh the risks...occurrences of rhabdomyolysis are extremely rare."[12]

Some abnormality is to be expected. Dr. Stephen Devries[13] wrote about liver issues in his book, *What Your Doctor May Not Tell You About Cholesterol.* If you want more information on cholesterol, I would highly recommend his book.

> Fortunately, the most severe side effect—actual muscle breakdown—is rare: about one out of five thousand for those taking the lowest doses and one out of two hundred for those taking the highest doses of statins. Very few people take the highest doses of satins. Very few people take the highest dose, estimated at less than 1 percent of those on statins. These patients tend to have extremely high cholesterol, so that the benefit of the medicine outweighs the side effects. In my nearly twenty years of experience with patients, I have never seen a single case of actual muscle breakdown. (153)

I have noticed that patients fret a great deal over potential liver abnormalities. Your liver is working too much if you have high LDL (bad) cholesterol. It needs to work less efficiently. People do very well if they work with their healthcare provider, keep appointments to get checkups, and report any side effects. You are at much higher risk for a heart attack or stroke if you do not get your LDL (bad) cholesterol down to safe levels.

Cost

Some statin drugs can be expensive. There are several different statins and many are available as a cheaper generic medication. If the cost is prohibitive, you do have options. Check with various pharmacies for a cheaper cost. You can ask your healthcare provider to prescribe a cheaper generic medication. You can also ask for a double dose and break it in half with a pill cutter. If you must take the more expensive medication, you can contact the pharmaceutical company that produced the medication and see if you qualify for a free supply.

Other Drugs to Lower LDL (Bad) Cholesterol

If you are in a high risk group and you can't tolerate the statin therapy or if you have high triglycerides, there are other medications that your healthcare provider could prescribe.

Takeaway Points

In summary, understanding your blood cholesterol can be summed up into one phrase, "Know your numbers and treat your risk category." Talk to your healthcare provider about your numbers. Are they under control? At a minimum, keep your LDL (bad) cholesterol below 100 mg/dL. However, if you fall into one of the four risk groups previously described, talk to your healthcare provider about cutting your baseline LDL (bad) cholesterol by half. Your pharmacist is another good resource regarding your medications.

After reading this chapter, I hope that you are ready to make a small change in your diet to reduce your risk for a heart attack or stroke. It is important information to understand the real culprit for heart disease: LDL (bad) cholesterol. Whether the source is genetics or diet, controlling LDL is the first step in halting plaque build-up. Eating less saturated fat will help, but medications are often required. If your healthcare provider wants you to take a statin, he or she has good reasons. Do your homework and ask many questions. The more that you eat a healthier diet, the less medication you will require.

Additional Information

American Heart Association   www.americanheart.org
American Stroke Association   www.strokeassociation.org
National Heart Lung and Blood Institute   www.nhlbi.org
Heart Attack Risk Calculator   https://www.heart.org/gglRisk/main_en_US.html
2013 Cholesterol Guidelines   http://circ.ahajournals.org/content/early/2013/11/11/01.cir.0000437738.63853.7a
USDA Myplate and Food Pyramid Resources   http://fnic.nal.usda.gov/dietary-guidance/myplatefood-pyramid-resources/usda-myplate-food-pyramid-resources

Drugs don't work in patients who don't take them.

—Former Surgeon General C. Everett Coop, MD

4

High Blood Pressure: The Silent Killer

High blood pressure, or hypertension, is a very dangerous and deadly problem. It is called the silent killer because most people are completely unaware that their blood pressure is too high, causing severe damage to their body. The statistics are startling. Nearly 30 percent of American adults have high blood pressure.[1] Of those, 75 percent are taking medications, but only 52 percent have it under control.[1] By age fifty-five, 90 percent of all adults will develop high blood pressure.[2]

If you have been told that your blood pressure is too high, this chapter will help you understand the danger that this silent threat imposes, how to detect if you have high blood pressure, and simple strategies to lessen its severity. If lifestyle changes are not enough, I will walk you through the common medications to lower blood pressure to safe levels.

Blood Pressure

Your blood pressure reading encompasses two numbers. The top number or systolic reading is a measurement of the pressure within the heart when it contracts. The bottom number or diastolic is a measurement of what the heart must pump against: the pressure in the aorta and the rest of the arteries.

Blood pressure fluctuates throughout the day based on the amount of adrenalin or epinephrine circulating within your system. Adrenalin is a powerful hormone that increases heart rate and blood pressure. It begins to surge in the early morning just prior to awaking and is the highest at midmorning. Waking up is stressful on the body, causing your blood pressure to rise. Throughout the rest of the day, blood pressure fluctuates and is at the lowest while you are sleeping. However, this pattern may be altered at night due to irregular sleeping patterns, nightmares, and sleep apnea. People stop breathing during sleep apnea episodes. Oxygen levels decrease triggering a release of adrenalin, which increases blood pressure. Sleep apnea is diagnosed with a sleep study.

Your blood pressure also increases with age. The average blood pressure of a newborn is 73/55, a child one month to five years old 95/75, a teenager 102/80, an adult and a healthy senior citizen 120/80, but may commonly increase to 160/95.[3]

Blood Pressure Measurement

There are several ways to measure a blood pressure. A cuff is placed around your upper arm and inflated so that arterial blood flow is blocked momentarily and the pulse in the arm is muted. Either a machine or a person listens for the sound of the return of the pulse and records that number as the top (systolic) one. While listening for the blood pressure sounds, the cuff is slowly deflated. When the pulse is no longer heard, the bottom (diastolic) number is recorded. Patiently listening for the sounds is a key component to obtaining an accurate blood pressure reading. Blood pressure is recorded as: Blood Pressure = _____/_____ mm Hg.

Adult Blood Pressure Levels

The word "hypertension" is the medical term for high blood pressure. In large studies, people have been evaluated across the globe to determine what levels of blood pressures lead to organ damage. You may visit www.nhlbi.gov to view a copy of the national guidelines and more information about this research and the rationale behind how the guidelines were developed.

Adult Blood Pressure Levels[2]

	Top Number (Systolic)	Bottom Number (Diastolic)
Normal Blood Pressure	Less than 120	Less than 80
Pre-high Blood Pressure (Pre-hypertension)	120-139	80-89
Stage 1 High Blood Pressure (Hypertension)	140-159	90-99
Stage 2 High Blood Pressure (Hypertension)	≥160	≥100
*Seventh Report of the Joint National Committee on Prevention, Detection, Evaluation & Treatment of High Blood Pressure (JNC 7)		

The most recent guidelines were released in 2014.[4] While many of the previous guidelines remained unchanged, some controversy has erupted. Previously, high blood pressure should be treated when numbers reached 140/90. Under the new guidelines if you are over fifty-nine years old, high blood pressure should be treated when it reaches 150/90. High blood pressure is so destructive that I agree with treatment beginning at levels of 140/90. I wanted you to be aware of this issue as specialists do not always agree when interpreting the science.

High Blood Pressure Classifications

Ideal blood pressure should be less than 120/80.[2] I know that number seems really low, but a great deal of research indicated that as numbers climb so does the damage and risk from higher pressures.

Pre-Hypertension

Pre-hypertension refers to blood pressures that fall between a top (systolic) number of 120 and 139 or a bottom (diastolic) number of 80 to 89.[2] The general recommendation for readings at this level is to engage in a healthier lifestyle and monitor your blood pressure. I will describe the lifestyle that lowers blood pressure and the frequency to monitor pre-hypertension blood pressures later within this chapter.

Stage 1 Hypertension

Any blood pressure that remains above either the top (systolic) number of 140 or the bottom (diastolic) number of 90 should be treated.[2] Lifestyle changes will help lower your blood pressure, but medications will be needed if you can't get both of those numbers under 140/90.

Stage 2 Hypertension

If your top (systolic) number is over 160 or if the bottom number is over 100, they are too high and must come down.[2] Although lifestyle changes are helpful, medications are usually needed to get the blood pressure to safe levels.

High Blood Pressure Emergencies

In some instances, rapid increases in blood pressure with very high readings requires a trip to the emergency room. These emergencies are triggered by adrenalin surges and are diagnosed with a blood pressure over 180/120.[2] Symptoms may include a severe headache, shortness of breath, nosebleeds, or severe anxiety.[2] Blood pressure this high can cause a stroke, so physicians will administer medication to drop it to safe levels. It is important to keep a record of your readings, and if they start to increase, contact your healthcare provider. If you are diagnosed with hypertension, have a discussion with your healthcare provider regarding the numbers that are considered worrisome.

Damage from High Blood Pressure

It is important to understand exactly how high pressure damages your body. As blood moves through the chambers of the heart, various valves keep it moving in one direction. When blood pressure is too high, the increased pressure causes the heart to work harder to pump blood into the aorta. The valves may become damaged and weakened. Ultimately, the valves may need to be replaced with open heart surgery. Treating high blood pressure protects the valves from further damage. In addition, the heart becomes enlarged and weaker from constantly pushing against the higher pressure in the aorta. Heart failure is a chronic condition that often follows years of uncontrolled high blood pressure.

Recall that in chapter 1, I described how your arteries should be smooth like the inside of your cheek. High pressure, much like sandpaper, causes a roughened surface within the inside lining of the arteries. The LDL (bad) cholesterol moving through the blood is caught within those rougher areas. Plaque begins to form and weakens the artery, which increases the risk for a heart attack or stroke.

End Organ Damage

Damage from high blood pressure occurs throughout all of the arteries of the body, causing other problems as well. In the eyes, it can lead to blindness, and in the kidneys, it causes kidney failure. The arteries are like tree branches that get smaller and smaller at the ends. The smallest arteries at the very ends of the arterial tree are blasted apart from the higher pressure. Once these vessels become permanently damaged, there are fewer arteries left to carry oxygen rich blood to the organs, which leads to end organ damage or organ failure. It takes a very large number of damaged vessels before symptoms occur. All organs may be affected. The real danger of high blood pressure is that the initial damage occurs without any symptoms. Tests can be done to check for end organ damage, but it is imperative to have blood pressure in a safe range to prevent additional damage.

Causes of High Blood Pressure

Primary Hypertension (High Blood Pressure)

In most cases, there is no explanation for high blood pressure. Many scientists believe that there is a strong genetic component as high blood pressure tends to run in families. It's also interesting that people may have normal blood pressure for many years and at some point blood pressures suddenly climb. Arteries are flexible and supple but become stiffer with age.

Lifestyle factors also increase your risk for high blood pressure. These include excess dietary salt intake, overweight, smoking, caffeine, alcohol, physical inactivity, stress, and a diet low in fruits and vegetables. Smoking cessation (chapter 7), weight loss (chapter 6), physical activity (chapter 8), and stress management (chapter 9) are covered in more detail in later sections of this book. Genetic variances also occur with some groups of people. African Americans have higher rates of high blood pressure than other groups.[1]

Secondary Hypertension (High Blood Pressure)

Some diseases increase your risk for chronic high blood pressure, but these are rare. They include kidney disease, problems with the aorta, tumors, hormonal disease, and rare neurological disorders. Some medications increase high blood pressure as well such as decongestants, ibuprofen, oral contraceptives, steroids, amphetamines, and cocaine.[2] Over-the-counter supplements may also raise blood pressure along with nicotine found within tobacco products. Interestingly, licorice is problematic. Always check with your healthcare provider or pharmacist about products that might raise your blood pressure.

Pregnancy

About 6 to 8 percent of pregnant women develop high blood pressure during pregnancy.[5] It can lead to complications for both the mother and the unborn child such as preeclampsia (high blood pressure), stroke, hemorrhage or acute liver and kidney problems. High blood pressure due to pregnancy is resolved once the baby is born.

Home Blood Pressure Monitoring

One abnormal reading does not lead to a diagnosis of hypertension. However, it is a red flag to gather more information. I tell my patients that you need to monitor your blood pressures at home to really help your healthcare provider determine whether or not you have high blood pressure. Was this reading an isolated finding? What happens after you eat a salty meal or you face a stressful event? Are they elevated when you are at home and relaxed?

Many people are in denial in regards to their high blood pressure. You feel good and just do not believe that damage is occurring. I encourage you to do some homework and monitor your blood pressure at home. If you remain in denial about your high blood pressure, your numbers will help move you into taking action to reduce the danger. It will help your healthcare provider with treatment decisions, but it must be done properly. Improper technique is a major problem within far too many health care offices.[6] If the cuff pressure is released too quickly, the higher numbers will not be heard and the value will be inaccurately low. As an example, I have high blood pressure. As a nursing professor, I taught proper technique to many nursing students. My pressures had been climbing, and I knew it was time to readjust my medication dosage. During an office visit, the nurse went too fast when taking the measurement and I knew that the reading would be inaccurate. She recorded 110/74. I asked her to check it again but much slower. Imagine her shock to hear it at 158/94. You should have seen her face. It certainly provided a teachable moment. Your home readings give your healthcare provider more accurate information.

White Coat Syndrome

White coat syndrome occurs in 20 percent of adults with high blood pressure.[7] It reflects a condition where blood pressure is normal at home but only high at the healthcare provider's office. It is important to remember that if your blood pressure is high in the doctor's office, it is probably high during other stressful times throughout the day as well. Tracking your numbers at home will provide your healthcare provider with a more accurate picture of your situation.

Blood Pressure Machine

While I haven't tried all of the machines on the market, I've had a great deal of experience with the automatic blood pressure machines for the upper arm. Each device is slightly different; however, follow the picture on the device and wrap the cuff around your bare arm as directed. I recommend that you sit for five minutes and then push the button to get the recording. You can buy these machines at many drugstores or big box stores, so shop around for the best price. You can visit http://www.bhsoc.org/default.stm or http://www.dableducational.org for recommendations for the most accurate devices. I would highly recommend that you buy a device that connects to power so that you don't have to buy batteries. If you do buy a battery-operated machine, be sure to get rechargeable batteries. The wrist and finger machines are less accurate and should be avoided.[7] Be aware that the public machines at pharmacies may not be well maintained and are often inaccurate as well.[7] If you have an irregular heartbeat such as atrial fibrillation, the machines will probably not record an accurate blood pressure.

Cuff Size

Be sure that you buy a blood pressure cuff that fits your arm properly. Use a tape measure around the middle section of your upper arm. The thigh area is only used when upper arms are not available for a blood pressure reading. I would encourage you to speak with you healthcare provider about which location is the most accurate for you to take your blood pressure.

Cuff Size Guidelines[8]

Arm Circumference	Cuff Size
8.5 to 10 inches	Small Adult
10.5 to 13 inches	Adult
13.5 to 17 inches	Large Adult
17.5 to 20 inches	Use Adult Thigh Cuff
*Blood Pressure: How Do You Measure Up? *Preventive Cardiovascular Nurses Association*	

Blood Pressure Technique and Recordings[7]

Empty your bladder before taking your blood pressure. Place the cuff on your non-dominant arm on a table at the level of your heart. For most people, it will be the left arm. Sit with your back against the chair with both feet on the floor for five minutes prior to obtaining the first reading. Push the button and record the number along with the date and time. Wait three minutes and take a second blood pressure. Readings may be taken again within as little as one minute, but I generally recommend three minutes between readings. Record the number. Check with your healthcare provider regarding how many readings you should take at one setting, but I think two are enough.

Take your blood pressure readings in the morning before you have any coffee, food, medications, or cigarettes and again at night prior to evening medications or going to bed. It is recommended that you follow this procedure on consecutive days for one week,[7] but I suggest that you do it for two weeks prior to your health care checkup. Note if this reading is occurring during times of stress, whether or not you ate a salty diet or forgot a blood pressure medication. My written log has helped me become more aware of the things that raise my blood pressure.

Blood Pressure Record

Date	Arm	Time	BP	Time	BP	Comments

Many people think that it is best to take blood pressure readings during times of stress or after exercise. The best information is gathered with the two-week approach. It will show your healthcare provider the range of both low and high blood pressures. During this two-week period, you should take a few readings in both arms, but normally, one arm will suffice. Your healthcare provider will want to see if you have large blood pressure differences between both arms. After you have completed the first two readings, move the cuff to the other arm, wait a few minutes, and repeat the cycle. You only need to do this one or two times during the two-week period. Use the arm with the highest readings for future blood pressure measurements.

In my experience, I have noticed that some people become very obsessive about their blood pressure readings. They record them several times throughout the day for weeks on end. You really do not have to take them any more often than previously described unless directed differently by your healthcare provider. Take your recordings and device to your appointment so that it can be checked for accuracy. Ask what numbers should cause alarm and require notification.

Treatment for High Blood Pressure

Lifestyle changes are the first step in reducing high blood pressure. However, if blood pressure is not controlled with these behavior changes, medications will be required. I begin this section with a description of the most helpful lifestyle changes and follow with common medications prescribed when lifestyle is not enough.

Lifestyle Changes to Lower Blood Pressure

The Trouble with Salt (Sodium)

Salt tastes good and has been used as a pleasant seasoning for thousands of years. However, the problem with salt or sodium is that wherever salt goes, water follows. If you eat a diet high in salt, the kidneys will retain water to help dilute the higher salt content in your blood. The excess fluid raises your blood pressure. Water pills or diuretics work by directing the kidneys to excrete salt. Water will follow and blood pressure will decrease.

If you eat a salty diet, you may require more medication to get rid of the excess water in order to reduce your blood pressure. It becomes a vicious cycle. Some people are very "salt sensitive." I'm one of them. If I eat a salty meal, my blood pressure will rise about two days later. Pay attention to how your blood pressure responds to your salt intake. Most of us will see a reduction in our blood pressures if we reduce the salt in our diet.

Americans enjoy eating out and partaking in junk food. Both are notoriously high in salt (sodium). The most recent 2013 national guidelines recommend that Americans ideally limit their salt intake to less than 1,500 mg/day.[9] Personally, I think these new salt restrictions are too difficult for most people to follow when you consider that the average American consumes on average 3,400 mg of sodium each day.[10] I remember caring for very sick patients with profound end stage heart failure drowning in excess fluid. Even modest increases in salt intake could put them in the hospital. Despite this dangerous situation, they had a very difficult time keeping their salt intake below 1,500 mg/day. However, any reduction in your salt intake will help to lower your blood pressure.

Reading a Food Label

Reducing the salt in your diet will not be easy. A good place to start is to become more familiar with the foods that are especially high in salt or sodium content.

Salt (Sodium) Content in Common Foods[11]

Food	Sodium (mg)
Roasted cured boneless ham	1,275
Cooked corned beef	964
Spaghetti sauce without meat (1/2 cup)	618
Salted pretzels (5 small twists)	486
Drained canned salmon	458
Cottage cheese, ½ cup (1%)	459
Processed lean roast beef (2 ounces)	440
French salad dressing (2 T)	428
1 (3 1/2") plain bagel	379
Apple pie 1/8 slice of 9" pie	333
Tortilla chips (1 ounce)	284
Corn flakes (1 cup)	240
Saltine crackers (5)	195
Cheddar cheese 1 ounce	176
1 slice white bread	135
Whole/skim milk (1 cup)	120
Baked chicken breast no skin (3 oz.)	63
1 egg	63
Baked salmon	56

Step by Step: Eating To Lower Your Blood Cholesterol
U.S. Department of Health and Human Services

The same strategy that you used in chapter 3 for reading the saturated fat content on a food label to make healthier choices will work for salt content as well. Check the sodium content on the label and try the food item that has the lowest amount of salt. Compare the sodium content of the following chips: Sea Salt Vinegar, Original Lightly Salted, and Unsalted. I think that you will be surprised how satisfied you will find the foods with the lower sodium content. They will certainly be much better for your blood pressure. I tried the unsalted product and was surprised. The crunchiness quenched my craving for a potato chip, and I didn't miss the salt as much as I thought that I would. Experimenting with different options is the goal here. Read and compare labels and try the lower sodium product.

Potato Chip Food Labels[12]

Sea Salt Vinegar		Original Lightly Salted		Unsalted	
Serving Size	(8 chips)	Serving Size	(8 chips)	Serving Size	(8 chips)
Calories/serving	140	Calories/serving	140	Calories/serving	130
Total fat	9 (g)	Total fat	9 (g)	Total fat	6 (g)
Saturated fat	1.5 (g)	Saturated fat	1.5 (g)	Saturated fat	1.5 (g)
Trans fat	0 (g)	Trans fat	0 (g)	Transfat	0 (g)
Cholesterol	0 (mg)	Cholesterol	0 (mg)	Cholesterol	0 (mg)
Sodium	380 (mg)	Sodium	110 (mg)	Sodium	0 (g)
Total carbohydrates	15 (g)	Total carbohydrates	15 (g)	Total carbohydrates	18 (g)
Dietary fiber	1 (g)	Dietary fiber	1 (g)	Dietary fiber	1(g)
Sugars	0 (g)	Sugars	0 (g)	Sugars	1 (g)
Protein	2 (g)	Protein	2 (g)	Protein	2 (g)

Remember that when you eat restaurant and fast food, it is generally very high in salt. Be mindful of this problem and try and reduce salt wherever you can.

Sodium Content in Restaurant Foods[11]

Fast Food	Sodium (mg)
Sub sandwich with cheese, salami, ham	1,650
Egg, cheese, bacon biscuit	1,261
Double patty cheeseburger with condiments	1,149
Pancakes with butter and syrup, 3	1,103
Chili con carne, 1 cup	1,008
Taco salad with chili, 1 1/2 cups	886
Grilled chicken sandwich, plain	758
Baked potato with cheese sauce & chili	701
Hot dog	671
Plain cheeseburger, single patty	500
Cheese pizza, 1/8 of 12"	336
Chocolate shake, 10 ounces	273
Step by Step: Eating To Lower Your Blood Cholesterol U. S. Department of Health and Human Services	

The Benefits of Fruits and Vegetables

The Dietary Approach to Stopping Hypertension (DASH) is a diet that is high in fruits and vegetables and lower in saturated fat and salt.[13] There are natural chemicals within fruits and vegetables such as potassium and magnesium that lower blood pressure. The DASH diet was studied to determine its effectiveness. The control group was adults eating a typical American diet high in saturated fats but low in fruits and vegetable intake. Another group received a diet high in saturated fats and salt but were given more fruits and vegetables. The third group was given the DASH diet, which was high in fruits and vegetables, lower in saturated fat and salt. The more fruits and vegetables consumed and less salt eaten, the greater reductions in blood pressure that were observed. Eating a plant-based diet provides many benefits that help maintain a healthy weight, improve cholesterol numbers, and lower blood pressure. Fill your plate with a colorful assortment of fruits and vegetables, eat less salt and saturated fat. Remember that any dietary change will begin to improve your blood pressure. Start with small, simple changes.

Weight Management

Excess weight is very hard on your blood pressure. Your body has to work harder to provide nutrients to the extra fat. "For every pound of fat, your body has to make several miles of blood vessels to keep it alive."[14] The extra weight is hard on the joints as well and causes many health problems. Even small amounts of weight loss improve blood pressure.[2] In chapter 6, I describe simple strategies that will help you lose weight and lower your blood pressure.

Smoking

With each puff on a cigarette, blood pressure increases due to an increase in adrenalin surge levels. The arteries are constantly bombarded with damaging toxic chemicals that are transported throughout the blood. Using any type of tobacco product causes many health problems. In chapter 7, I spend a great deal of time describing strategies that have worked for other smokers who quit. Blood pressure improves immediately with cessation.

Caffeine

Drinking more than four cups of coffee a day increases blood pressure and risk for a heart attack and stroke.[15] Caffeine is found in coffee, tea, soft drinks, chocolate, other foods, medications, and supplements.

Amount of Caffeine in Common Foods[16]

Fast Food	Caffeine (mg)
Starbucks Coffee, tall (12 fluid oz.)	260
5-Hour Energy (1.9 fluid oz.)	208
NoDoz or Vivarin 1 caplet	200
Excedrine Migraine 2 tablets	130
Red Bull (8.4 fluid oz.)	80
Snapple Lemon Tea (16 fluid oz.)	62
Mountain Dew, regular or diet (12 oz.)	54
Cold Stone Creamery Mocha Ice Cream (12 fluid oz.)	52
Jolt Gum 1 piece	45
Coca-Cola, Coke Zero, Diet Pepsi (12 oz.)	35
Hershey's Cocoa 1 Tbs.	8
*Caffeine Content of Food and Drugs *Center for Science in the Public Interest*	

In addition, the US Food and Drug Administration issued a warning against the use of "caffeine powder."[17] The powder is sold as a dietary supplement. One teaspoon contains as much caffeine as twenty-five cups of coffee.

> Very small amounts may cause accidental overdose…it is almost impossible to accurately measure powdered pure caffeine with normal kitchen measuring tools…anyone with a heart condition should not use the powder.

Healthy Coping with Afternoon Fatigue

In the afternoon, you may begin to feel sluggish and sleepy. If you can't take a nap, there are a few other strategies that you might try before pouring yourself another cup of coffee. Some fatigue is related to dehydration. I was never very good at drinking water, but if I poured a glass from the office cooler and left it on my desk, I found that I drank it in between phone calls and work. Rather than reaching for a high calorie caffeinated soda, try a can of sparkling water. Movement helps too. Get out of your chair, move around, or place your head down while touching your toes. The blood moving to your brain increases oxygen and will help wake you up.

Alcohol

Too much alcohol raises blood pressure. The national guidelines for the treatment of high blood pressure recommend no more than two drinks a day for men and one drink a day for women.[2] One drink is equal to 12 ounces of beer, 5 ounces of wine or 1.5 ounces of liquor.

Physical Activity

Being more active works like a pill to lower your blood pressure. When you begin to exercise, blood moves from your core organs out to the working muscles to increase oxygen and energy. Recall that oxygen is needed to make energy to do any type of work. This movement of blood actually lowers your blood pressure. In addition, exercise increases your metabolism rate for hours after the exercise has ceased, burning calories and fat. In chapter 8, I describe simple ways to add activities that are fun into your life, which will help lower your blood pressure. Remember that all activities count.

Stress

Stress increases your blood pressure due a surge in your adrenalin. In chapter 9, I describe several strategies to help you reduce and manage your stress, which will help lower your blood pressure.

Medications to Lower Blood Pressure

If lifestyle changes do not bring your blood pressure down to safe levels, medications will be needed. The goal of treatment is a blood pressure below 140/90.[2] However, for people with a history of a heart attack or stroke, diabetes, or kidney disease, the goal will be less than 130/80.[2] You should speak with your healthcare provider for your individual goal based on your medical condition.

Several different classes of medications can be prescribed to treat high blood pressure.[4] It may take several adjustments to get the right medication and dose for each individual patient. Tracking your blood pressure at home as previously described will help your healthcare provider understand how you are responding to the prescribed treatment. The following list covers some of the more commonly prescribed medications. Please remember that your healthcare provider knows your medical condition best and may have other medications or combinations of medications that are beyond this list. Your pharmacist is another great resource.

ACE Inhibitors[18]

ACE inhibitors such as captopril, enalapril, lisinopril lower blood pressure by interrupting a chemical process that constricts the arteries, which leads to higher blood pressures. Most people tolerate this class of antihypertensive medication very well, but dizziness and fatigue may occur if the blood pressure is lowered too much. A dry cough may develop in some people. These drugs should not be taken during pregnancy as it may harm the unborn baby.

Angiotensin Receptor Blockers[18]

Angiotensin receptor blockers such as eprosartan, candesartan, losartan, valsartan, and irbesartan lower blood pressure by blocking a chemical reaction that constricts the arteries. As with any hypertensive, dizziness and fatigue can occur from lowering the blood pressure too much. Some people may experience a sore throat, runny nose, joint discomfort, or abdominal pain. The complication of a cough is much less with this medication than the ACE Inhibitors. These drugs should not be taken during pregnancy as it may harm the unborn baby.

Beta-Blockers[18]

Beta-blocker medications such as atenolol and metoprolol block the effects of the hormone adrenalin. When you are under stress, adrenalin surges increase your heart rate and blood pressure. The blocking effect slows the heart rate and helps the heart contract less forcefully. In addition, the blood vessels dilate, which allows oxygen to flow more freely to the heart and other organs. The medication should never be stopped abruptly. Common side effects are dizziness and fatigue from lowering the blood pressure too much, a heart rate that is too slow, diarrhea, and decreased libido. Notify your healthcare provider if you have a history of asthma as beta-blockers can make it worse.

Calcium Channel Blockers[18]

Calcium channel blockers such as amlodipine, diltiazem, and nitrendipine cause the smooth muscle inside the lining of the artery to relax or dilate, which lowers blood pressure. Side effects may include dizziness and fatigue from lowering your blood pressure too much. Some people may have increased edema or swelling of the lower legs, and headaches.

Thiazide-Type Diuretics[18]

The common name for a diuretic is "water pill." There are several different types of diuretics such as bendroflumethiazide, chlorthalidone, indapamide, and furosemide, but they basically work in the same way. They direct the kidney to excrete more sodium (salt). Wherever salt goes, water follows. As the water is excreted, important electrolytes or chemicals such as potassium are excreted. It's important to have these electrolytes checked by your healthcare provider to ensure that you are not losing too much. In many cases, potassium may need to be supplemented. Weakness, headache, and abdominal discomfort are some side effects that have been reported. However, most people tolerate these medications very well.

Other Medication Issues to Consider

Antihypertensives work to lower blood pressure. It is imperative to monitor blood pressure at home and keep appointments so that your healthcare provider may have an accurate picture of your treatment response. Remember to rise slowly from sitting positions to avoid fainting because blood pools in your lower legs when you sit for prolonged periods of time. If you rise too quickly, blood will remain in your lower legs and not get into your head fast enough. It takes the blood a few seconds longer to readjust to a change in your position. Hot baths may lower blood pressures too much as well. The hot temperatures lead to pooling of blood in the extremities away from your brain. Dizziness may ensue. Extreme heat may also lead to heat exhaustion. It is harder for the body to cool when you are taking some blood pressure medications. If you are ill, monitor your blood pressure and notify your healthcare provider for values that are either too high or too low. You may need an adjustment in your medication. Dehydration from diarrhea and vomiting are potentially problematic.

The benefits of treatment far outweigh the risks of no treatment of high blood pressure. It is important to work as a team with your healthcare provider to control high blood pressure with the least amount of side effects. Report any problems immediately. I've noticed that people sometimes give up treatment if the first medication used doesn't get the job done. The National Community of Pharmacists sponsored a survey of 1,000 adults in 2006 and reported that 49 percent had forgotten to take their prescribed medication, 31 percent had not filled their prescription, 24 percent had taken less than the recommended dose, and 10 percent substituted an over-the-counter supplement instead of taking the prescription given to them.[19] Other researchers found that people stop taking their cholesterol medications after six months.[20]

In chapter 10, I describe a variety of strategies that you can employ to overcome personal medication barriers. If you can't get it done with healthier habits, medication will be needed. However, if you are someone who is living a very healthy lifestyle and you still have elevated numbers, then you have inherited a propensity for high blood pressure. You may need medication to counter your genetic vulnerability. Don't get discouraged. Since you are doing so many things well, you will not require as much medication as someone who has a similar genetic makeup but making poor lifestyle choices. Learn as much as you can about the aspects of your treatment plan. Ask many questions and work as a team with your healthcare provider and pharmacist. The goal is to reduce your risk so that you may live a longer healthier life.

Personal Story

My blood pressures were normal until I went through menopause. Then it was like a time bomb went off, and all of a sudden, my blood pressures were dangerously high. The first clue that there was a problem was an elevated blood pressure reading during a routine physical: white coat syndrome. Like many of you, I just didn't want to believe that I suddenly had a problem that needed medication to control. Even though I was educated about high blood pressure, I remained in denial. A nurse friend chided me,

"Jennie, do you want to have a stroke? Take the medicine. You know better." Of course, she was right.

I'm on three medications now to counter my genetic vulnerability as both of my parents had high blood pressure. I've learned that a healthy lifestyle is important and allows me to require less medication. Controlling high blood pressure takes a great deal of teamwork with my doctor to ensure that my numbers remain at safe levels. Recently, we increased the dose of one of my blood pressure pills. I didn't see it as a failure but rather an opportunity to enjoy a longer and healthier life.

Takeaway Points

High blood pressure is the leading cause of stroke.[1] It also silently damages all of the arteries of the body and profoundly increases risk for a heart attack. It is vital to work with your healthcare provider to keep it below 140/90. While a healthy lifestyle is key, medications are often needed. My story highlights the challenge of managing high blood pressure. Even experts have a hard time following their own advice. Listen to your healthcare provider and work as a team. It isn't always easy to control your blood pressure, but you can do it!

Additional Information

National Heart, Lung and Blood Institute   www.nhlbi.gov
American Heart Association   www.americanheart.org
Heart 360   https://www.heart360.org/
Preventive   Cardiovascular   Nurses   Association   (PCNA)
    http://pcna.net/patients—preventive-cardiovascular-nurses-association

Failure is not fatal, but failure to change might be.

—College Basketball Coach, John Wooden

5

The Danger from Diabetes

Of all the cardiovascular risk factors, I think that diabetes is the most difficult to manage. Whatever a person with diabetes eats or doesn't eat will alter his or her blood sugar. They have to think about it twenty-four hours each and every day for the rest of their lives. If blood sugars aren't under control, the excess sugar causes extensive damage throughout the body, which impairs quality and length of life.

In this chapter, I want to encourage you to act now before you become a diabetic statistic. Believe me, you don't want to get this disease! As you look into the window of the life of a person with diabetes, perhaps you will be motivated to change your behaviors to avoid this destructive disease. If you already have diabetes, you will be reminded of the importance of managing your blood sugars in order to prevent the common complications such as blindness, kidney failure, a heart attack, or stroke. This chapter is included in my book because most persons with diabetes die from cardiovascular-related problems.[1] Consider this chapter your wake-up call to really think about how you are taking care of your body. Hopefully, you will have an understanding of this deadly disease and the simple things that you can do to lower blood sugar and reduce your risk.

Overview of Diabetes

The number of American adults diagnosed with diabetes number 19.7 million.[1] Tragically, another 8.2 million are unaware that they have the disease. There are approximately 87.3 million or 38 percent of American adults who have pre-diabetes.[1] Not all pre-diabetics will develop diabetes, but this condition causes harm throughout the body and is a great risk for other health problems. The incidence of diabetes is an epidemic that appears to be expanding along with the obesity epidemic. Between 1980 and 1990, approximately 5.5 percent of the US population was diagnosed with the disease, but by 2010, it had almost doubled, including 9.3 percent of all adults.[2]

Normal Blood Sugar Metabolism

Normally, after eating a meal, food is digested and enters the bloodstream as glucose or blood sugar. The organ called the pancreas detects the higher sugar in the blood and immediately releases a hormone called insulin. Think of insulin as the chemical key that unlocks the cell door to let sugar in to be used by the body. Your body combines the sugars from digested food with oxygen to create energy to keep you alive. More food produces greater amounts of blood sugar and stimulates the pancreas to secrete more insulin. When everything is working well, insulin and blood sugar levels rise and fall with your changing food intake and energy expenditure.

The Role of Insulin

Insulin levels rise sharply within a few minutes of eating, peak within 45 minutes and then drift back to the pre-meal baseline level. The speed which blood sugar rises depends upon the type of food that you eat. Carbohydrates, which are sugars and starches such as breads, desserts, and juices are easily broken down and enter the bloodstream very quickly. Fresh fruits and vegetables are higher in fiber and take longer to digest, slowing the time it takes to enter the bloodstream. Vegetables take longer to break down compared to fruits. Proteins such as meats and nuts are still longer while fats take the longest to breakdown. Persons with diabetes must rely on this information to plan meals and medications.

I do not counsel persons with diabetes regarding their diet as I think that is best left up to diabetes experts. It takes specially trained and experienced nurse and dietitian educators to counsel patients regarding their food choices and medications. If you have diabetes, I would refer you to the American Diabetes Association and your healthcare provider for information on learning how to manage your disease. However, in chapter 6, I describe strategies to stabilize blood sugar levels in order to reduce cravings and successfully manage weight. You might find that chapter helpful as well.

The Types of Diabetes

There are three types of diabetes: type 1 diabetes, type 2 diabetes, and gestational diabetes.

Type 1 Diabetes

Type 1 diabetes used to be known as juvenile diabetes or insulin-dependent diabetes type I. The terminology was simplified to "type 1 diabetes." It accounts for less than 5 percent to 10 percent of all cases of diabetes.[1] It generally develops in childhood, adolescence, or young adulthood, but it can occur at any time in life. For reasons unknown, the pancreas is literally destroyed. All insulin production stops. Many believe that some people with type 1 diabetes have inherited a genetic problem that makes them vulnerable to a virus that attacks and destroys the pancreas. Food eaten is broken down into blood sugar, but is unable to enter the cells because insulin is not available to unlock the door. The sugar remains in the blood. People who have type 1 diabetes are often very thin because their tissues are starving. The sugar is not getting to where it belongs. The excess sugar in the blood profoundly damages all of their arteries and organs. This situation is very dangerous and needs immediate correction. If not treated with medication, type 1 diabetes is fatal.

Treatment for Type 1 Diabetes

The person with type 1 diabetes will need insulin replacement injections several times a day for the rest of their life. In addition, they will need to prick their fingers with a needle several times throughout the day to measure their blood sugar levels. In general, this occurs prior to all meals and snacks, occasionally after meals, at bedtime, prior to exercise, before driving, or when they suspect a low blood sugar.[3] If an abnormal blood sugar reading is too high, insulin must be administered. If the reading is too low, sugar must be ingested. Insulin management is difficult because it is like walking a tightrope—too much and the heart may stop, too little and coma may result.

Risk Factors of Type 1 Diabetes

While there are not many risk factors for type 1 diabetes, family history or genetic vulnerabilities seem to play a role. If type 1 diabetes is found in a family, it is recommended that all family members be tested for the disease and genetic vulnerabilities.[3]

Type 1 diabetes attacks young people like a thief in the night. It comes on very suddenly so prevention isn't much of an option. However, if you have the disease, there is much that can be done to manage it. As technology advances, new methods for testing are being developed to avoid the multiple daily finger pricks required to measure blood sugar.

Insulin pumps are small machines that deliver insulin continuously. An extra dose of insulin may be needed prior to meals and when blood sugar levels are too high. A catheter is inserted into the fatty tissue of the upper torso and left in for a few days before it is removed and a new one inserted. It avoids the need for several injections a day. Pancreas/kidney transplant surgery is available if an organ and a donor match can be found, but few persons with type 1 diabetes are able to utilize this procedure.

Personal Story

I had a coworker who managed her type 1 diabetes better than any person with diabetes that I have ever met. She was highly educated and motivated about controlling her disease for over thirty years. However, even with her disciplined management, at times, she would go into a hypoglycemic reaction with dangerously low blood sugar levels and never really know why. This dangerous situation may result in life-threatening complications as blood sugar levels plummet. The brain is damaged and the heart may go into a lethal rhythm, which can result in death. Anyone taking insulin has to be watchful for this potentially deadly complication.

My purpose in describing type 1 diabetes in such detail is that insulin management is difficult and painful. If persons with type 2 diabetes do not control their blood sugar, they may worsen and also need to take insulin. While there isn't much that can be done to prevent type 1 diabetes, there is a great deal that can be done to prevent type 2 diabetes and the need for insulin.

Type 2 Diabetes

Type 2 diabetes is the most common type and makes up 90 percent to 95 percent of all cases.[1] It was called noninsulin dependent type II diabetes or adult onset diabetes for many years. The name was simplified to "type 2 diabetes." Lifestyle habits play a very large role in the development of the disease. There is a long period of time where blood sugar levels begin to rise before it reaches a level to be diagnosed as type 2 diabetes.[3] The good news is that early detection and interventions can halt the progression of the disease. The bad news is that most people are completely unaware of their elevated blood sugar levels until a great deal of damage has occurred.[1]

Insulin Resistance

Type 2 diabetes begins with a condition called "insulin resistance." It is a medical term that means the insulin present is not working very well. The cells or tissues of the body are not letting the sugar into the cell as readily as it should. Sometimes, the insulin drives the sugar into the cell, and other times, it doesn't work. Over time, less and less insulin is effective. The cells become "resistant" to insulin. The insulin may be present, but the cells are not responding to it any more.

The Connection with Excess Weight

Genetics play a role because type 2 diabetes tends to run in families. However, excess weight and inactivity play an even larger role. Each time that you eat excess calories, your pancreas has to work very hard to make enough insulin to lower your blood sugar. The body stores much of the excess sugar as fat. In the earliest stages, there is an increase in insulin secretion. It's hard to guess how much insulin will be needed and excess amounts may remain circulating in the blood after the meal is consumed.

In simplest terms, when you take in excess calories, your pancreas has to make much more insulin to handle those extra calories. Eventually, the pancreas wears out and can no longer do its job. At that point, blood sugar levels rise and you become a person with type 2 diabetes. It all started with excess caloric intake and lack of physical activity.

Treatment for Type 2 Diabetes

The primary treatment for Type 2 diabetes is lifestyle changes. Maintaining a healthy body weight will reduce the workload placed on the pancreas. Physical activity burns up the excess blood sugar for energy so that less insulin is required. However, lifestyle changes are difficult to maintain for many people. When lifestyle isn't enough, oral medications can be prescribed to help the pancreas work more efficiently. Some persons with type 2 diabetes will lose enough pancreas function and will need insulin injections with frequent blood glucose monitoring.[3]

Risk Factors of Type 2 Diabetes

Genetic vulnerabilities, obesity, and a lack of regular physical activity are large risk factors and have been previously discussed. For reasons not completely understood, Native Americans, Hispanics, and African Americans have higher rates of diabetes. Low (HDL) good cholesterol (below 35) and high triglycerides (above 150) often precede type 2 diabetes.[4] Women who gave birth to babies who weighed more than nine pounds are at greater risk as well. A recording of any elevated fasting blood sugar above 100 is a red flag that diabetes may be imminent if lifestyle changes are not started. Medications or supplements may also increase blood sugars. Always check with your healthcare provider or pharmacist for any potential side effects. If you have any of these characteristics, it is important to monitor and manage your blood sugar levels with diet, exercise, and medications if necessary. It is imperative to work with your healthcare provider to monitor the progression of the disease and response to treatment.

Gestational Diabetes

Gestation is the medical term for pregnancy. Pregnancy places a great strain on a mother's body. Gestational diabetes occurs in 2 percent to 10 percent of all pregnancies.[1] There is a problem in how the mother's body breaks down carbohydrates and blood sugar levels rise. As the pregnancy progresses, greater amounts of insulin are required. It is thought that the maternal hormones are responsible for elevated blood sugar levels during pregnancy. Gestational diabetes runs in families and is a leading risk factor for developing type 2 diabetes later in life.[1] Mothers with gestational diabetes are at greater risk for preterm labor and stillbirth. Babies may be larger than normal, making delivery more difficult. The excess blood sugar from the mother is delivered to the unborn baby especially at birth. Prior to birth, the baby compensates and produces additional insulin, which may cause problems due to low blood sugar. Maternal blood sugar levels that are too high or too low may impact growth and development within the unborn baby. Fetal distress during birth and respiratory complications following birth are not uncommon. Gestational diabetes is resolved with the birth of the baby. All pregnant women should be tested for elevated blood sugar levels between twenty-four and twenty-eight weeks of pregnancy.[3]

Risk Factors of Gestational Diabetes

Managing weight gain, increasing physical activity, and regular prenatal checkups are important to ensure that the blood sugar remains at healthy levels. Mothers with elevated blood sugar will need to monitor their levels daily throughout their pregnancy. Insulin may be needed to keep blood sugar levels under control.

Prevention of Gestational Diabetes

Genetic vulnerabilities, obesity, and lack of physical activity seem to be large risk factors for gestational diabetes. Pregnant women older than thirty years are at greater risk.[3] Any sign of an elevated fasting blood sugar level above 100 or signs of sugar in the urine is a special concern. Keep your weight under control, eat more fruits and vegetables, and take a twenty-minute walk each day. These simple strategies will provide major health benefits for you and your baby.

Complications from Diabetes

Elevated blood sugar levels cause damage to the arteries and organs throughout the body. The medical term for the damage to the smaller tiny vessels is called microvascular damage while the damage to the larger vessels is called macrovascular damage.

Small Artery Damage (Microvascular)

Eyes (Retinopathy)

The eyes are very sensitive to changes in the blood supply. In diabetes, the tiny vessels at the very ends of the branches become damaged. Eventually, vision will be impacted. Blindness and eye problems occur in 29 percent of persons with diabetes.[2] Annual dilated eye exams by and experienced ophthalmologist or optometrist are vital to detect early changes.[3]

Kidneys (Nephropathy)

Diabetes causes 44 percent of all cases of kidney failure in the United States.[2] Persons with diabetes often have high blood pressure, which also increases the kidney damage. The tiny vessels become broken and protein begins to abnormally leak into the urine. A twenty-four-hour urine test measures the amount of protein leakage and is often the first indicator of a problem. A glomerular filtration rate test measures how well the kidneys are filtering waste products. Lower numbers indicate poorer kidney function. When kidney failure is profound, dialysis may be required. Dialysis is a very time-consuming, invasive, and uncomfortable procedure. You are connected to a machine that replaces the function of the kidneys. Your blood moves through the machine, which filters the waste products from the blood. Typically, patients require dialysis three times a week for several hours a session.

Nerves (Neuropathy)

As the tiny vessels are damaged, nerves are also impacted. These problems may also lead to abnormal sweating, sudden low blood pressure drops when standing, bladder problems, sexual dysfunction, and gastrointestinal issues. It is important to get up slowly to allow the blood pressure to readjust to the change in position in order to prevent dizziness.

Large Artery Damage (Macrovascular)

Whenever blood sugar level is elevated, excess sugar scratches and damages the inside lining of the arteries and veins. The LDL (bad) cholesterol can get caught in those damaged areas. High blood pressure is present in the majority of persons with diabetes.[3] It is for this reason that heart disease is the leading cause of death.[1] Persons with diabetes are twice as likely to get a heart attack and stroke as persons without diabetes.[1] You can review chapter 1 for how this process occurs.

Poor Wound Healing

Recurrent infections are another complication from diabetes. The excess sugar provides a rich environment for harmful bacteria to grow. Infection fighters such as white blood cells have a harder time getting to the infected areas. Wounds take longer to heal, which may result in gangrene and the risk for an amputation. Some people may experience itching, visual disturbances, and symptoms related to organ damage of the kidneys and nerves. It is imperative that persons with diabetes keep their blood sugar, blood pressure, and LDL (bad) cholesterol low.

Diagnosis of Diabetes

Symptoms of Diabetes

Although many people are unaware of their elevated blood sugar levels, there are three cardinal symptoms that may indicate that something is wrong: frequent urination, unquenchable thirst, and insatiable hunger. The kidneys try to correct the excess blood sugar by expelling more sugar in the urine. Water is eliminated along with the sugar and urination is more frequent. Losing water will stimulate the thirst center in the brain and you will feel thirsty. Even though there is plenty of sugar in the blood, it is not getting into your tissues or cells. You feel like you are starving, and in reality, your tissues are starving. Your brain is telling you to increase your food intake, but even if you eat more food, it is not helping your body. The sugar is unusable to the body. You feel fatigued, due to a malnourished state. These symptoms occur in very lean persons with type 1 diabetes as well as in obese people who have type 2 diabetes. Nausea and vomiting from the abnormal breakdown of fat and muscle may also occur.

Blood Tests to Diagnosis Diabetes

Diabetes is diagnosed with an eight-hour fasting blood sugar test, an oral glucose tolerance test, and a hemoglobin A1C test.

Diabetes Diagnostic Blood Test Levels[3]

	Fasting Blood Sugar Test (8 hours)	2 Hour Oral Glucose Tolerance Test	Hemoglobin A1C Test
Normal	Less than 100 mg/dl	Less than 140 mg/dl	Less than 5.7%
Pre-diabetes	100 to 125 mg/dl	140 to 199 mg/dl	5.7% to 6.4%
Diabetes	Greater than 125 mg/dl	Greater than 199 mg/dl	Greater than 6.5%
*American Diabetes Association			

Fasting Eight-Hour Blood Sugar Test

Overnight fasting levels reflect how much sugar the liver is secreting while you sleep. A normal test is less than 101, a pre-diabetes level is between 101 and 125, while a diabetes level is over 125 and may indicate a problem.[3] Diabetes guidelines suggest that if a blood sugar is elevated, repeat the test.

Oral Glucose Tolerance Test (OGTT)

An oral glucose tolerance test (OGTT) is recommended when an abnormal random non-fasting test is elevated. It is a more specific and accurate test of how well the body breaks down sugar. It measures the ability of the pancreas to secrete insulin and the cells ability to respond to the insulin. A certain amount of sugar is given followed by a blood sugar test exactly two hours later. A normal person should be able to digest the dietary sugar and have normal blood sugar levels after two hours. Someone with pre-diabetes will have a blood sugar level between 140 to 199 while someone with diabetes will be over 199.[3]

Hemoglobin A1C

The fasting blood sugar test and the oral glucose tolerance test measures your blood sugar at a certain point in time. The hemoglobin A1C test measures your blood sugar over a period of 90 to 120 days. This test measures how much sugar attached to the red blood cells in that time frame. Higher levels of sugar in the blood will cause more sugar to attach to the red blood cells and the test will have higher results. The amount detected gives the healthcare provider an idea of how well controlled your blood sugars were over the life of the red blood cell. A normal reading is less than 5.7 percent, pre-diabetes is between 5.7 percent to 6.4 percent, while diabetes is more than 6.5 percent.[3] The treatment goals are set by your healthcare provider.

All adults over the age of forty-five should be screened at least every three years for diabetes.[3] Any adult who is overweight or has additional risk factors for diabetes should be tested as well.[3] Children ten years of age or older who are overweight or have two or more risk factors for diabetes should also be screened.[3]

Lifestyle Changes and Diabetes

Diabetes Prevention Trial

The Diabetes Prevention Trial studied 1,079 obese people who had pre-diabetes and were at a greater risk for converting to type 2 diabetes.[5] The participants were recruited from twenty-seven centers across the United States and were followed on average for 3 years.[5] One group received the diabetes prevention medication

Metformin. This medication reduces the amount of sugar released from the liver, absorbed from the intestine, and helps the fat cells utilize blood sugar more efficiently.[6] Another group received a placebo drug and a third group engaged in an intensive lifestyle intervention program with personal counseling. The intensive lifestyle group was required to attend a sixteen-week program, encouraged to eat a healthier diet, walk 150 minutes a week, and lose 7 percent of their body weight. As an example, a 200-pound person would be encouraged to lose 14 pounds during the three-year period.

The medication and lifestyle group were compared to the group that didn't get either intervention. Throughout the study, blood sugars were measured among other things. The researchers were looking for the number of persons with pre-diabetes who converted to type 2 diabetes. At the conclusion of the study, the group that received Metformin reduced their risk for developing type 2 diabetes by 31 percent.[5] However, the lifestyle intervention group decreased their risk by 58 percent.[5] Lifestyle changes were more powerful than the medication Metformin.

This study demonstrated how important lifestyle changes are to improving health. Eating a healthier diet not only improves your blood sugar numbers but it also helps you to control your weight. Losing just a small amount of weight and simple exercises, such as walking, help to maintain normal blood sugar levels. Using a lifestyle coach helps enhance motivation. If you are unable to make healthy lifestyle changes, your healthcare provider will have to correct your abnormal blood sugar levels with medication.

Medications and Diabetes

Insulin

Insulin is needed for all persons with type 1 diabetes and some persons with type 2 diabetics.[3] Recall that insulin is the chemical key that unlocks the cell door to let the sugar in to make energy. The amount of insulin needed varies with the amount and type of food that is eaten. There are various forms of insulin that peak at different time points such as rapid-acting, intermediate, and long-acting injection forms.

The challenge is to match the amount of insulin needed with the amount of food eaten. Too little insulin and the blood sugar remains high, damaging the arteries. Too much insulin and the blood sugar is lowered to dangerous levels, causing harm to the brain or triggering a lethal heart rhythm abnormality.

Low Blood Sugar (Hypoglycemia)

Hypoglycemia is a dangerous complication wherein insulin drives blood sugars to critically low levels. Symptoms include: unusual sweating, feeling faint or shaky, impaired vision, hunger, irritability, personality change, trouble thinking, or awakening. It can result in shock, unconsciousness, and cardiac arrest. Blood sugar levels must be raised immediately! The brain needs sugar in order to function. Serious complications begin when blood sugars are lower than 50.[3] While it occurs more frequently in persons with type 1 diabetes, it may also occur in persons with type 2 diabetes who take insulin. You must work closely with your healthcare provider to know when you should be concerned with low blood sugar levels and the appropriate treatments to correct it.

High Blood Sugar (Hyperglycemia/Ketoacidosis)

If insulin treatment is inefficient, an opposite reaction may occur where blood sugar levels are dangerously too high. This condition is called hyperglycemia or ketoacidosis. The very high blood sugar levels can lead to a diabetic coma. When your cells do not get the glucose that they need, the body breaks down muscle and fat. This breakdown creates fatty acids or ketones that enter the blood. The kidneys try to compensate by eliminating the harmful ketones, but they are not successful. The ketones that are not removed eventually poison the body, which leads to the coma. Symptoms may include: severe thirst, frequent urination, large amounts of sugar and ketones in the urine, labored breathing, nausea and vomiting, fruity-smelling breath, fatigue, and coma.[7] This dangerous disorder may be caused by many things that raise blood sugar levels such as infections, the stress of surgery, alcohol abuse, trauma, or other serious medical events.

Oral Medications

Oral medications are not effective in persons with type 1 diabetes who are dependent upon insulin. However, there are several medications that may help correct some of the blood sugar abnormalities found among persons with type 2 diabetes. Typically, the medications help the pancreas produce more insulin or make the tissues more responsive to its effects. The healthcare provider examines each individual situation to prescribe the appropriate medication.

Most problematic is that as blood sugar enters the cells, nutrition is improved and weight gain may be a common problem. While medications are very helpful, nothing takes the place of a small amount of weight loss, a healthier diet, and some physical activity to improve blood sugar levels. The more you are able to do with lifestyle changes, the less medication that you will need. Ultimately, the choice is up to you. Preventing diabetes in the first place is the primary goal.

The Metabolic Syndrome and Pre-Diabetes

Metabolic Syndrome

The metabolic syndrome represents a cluster of symptoms that indicate a problem with how your body is beginning to handle blood sugar. You do not have diabetes yet, but you are heading in that direction. If you have three out of the five of these clinical symptoms, you are said to have the disorder. The symptoms of the metabolic syndrome include[4]

- Blood pressure greater than 130/85.
- HDL (good) cholesterol less than 40 for men and less than 50 for women.
- Fasting triglycerides greater than 150.
- Fasting blood sugar equal to or greater than 100.
- Waist circumference greater than 40 inches for men or greater than 35 inches for women.

The metabolic syndrome may be present with a normal blood sugar. This cluster of symptoms is a warning that something is wrong and you need to make a correction or diabetes, a heart attack, or stroke may occur. The combination of low HDL (good) cholesterol and high triglycerides is especially problematic and may precede diabetes as well.

Pre-Diabetes

Pre-diabetes is diagnosed with a fasting blood sugar level between 100 and 125.[3] You should view pre-diabetes as a dangerous red flag. Your arteries are being damaged with each rise in blood sugar, and now is the time to take this condition seriously. The treatment begins with lifestyle changes of a healthy diet, weight loss, and increased physical activity. Medications may also be needed to block the progression of the disease.

Celebrities with Diabetes

Just as with the discussion of heart attacks and strokes in chapter 2, I think that it is helpful to learn from others who have lived with a particular disease, in this case diabetes.

Celebrities with Type 1 Diabetes

Mary Tyler Moore (Golden Globe–Winning Actress)[8]

The seventy-two-year-old actress Mary Tyler Moore was diagnosed with type 1 diabetes at thirty-two years old at the height of her career. In an interview, she stated:

> It is a fact of life that if someone invites you out to dinner you have to think, "What are they going to be doing when they serve you dinner? How quickly are they going to get it on the table from the time I arrive? When should I take my shot? What should I eat of what's available?" I shoot myself right through my clothes there at the table, right here in my thigh. I seldom wear white as a result.

Moore is the International Chairwomen for the Juvenile Diabetes Research Foundation. She says that the secret to her blood sugar control has been regular exercise. She works out five to six times per week for an hour on a treadmill. She has visual impairments but states that there have only been a few blips along the way. "I must say, I did a remarkable job of it." Moore looks great for battling this devastating disease for so many years.

Jay Cutler (Chicago Bears, Quarterback)[9]

Cutler was diagnosed with type 1 diabetes in 2008. He was twenty-four years old at the height of his professional football career. Cutler described his experience with diabetes.

Diabetes is all about insulin levels and sugar levels and what you put in your body. The more you put in your body the more you have to regulate it with insulin. So later kickoffs you're talking about breakfast, lunch and a pregame meal, so that's more food you've got to be aware of and what you put in your body. A noon game, light breakfast, a little fruit and some insulin and I'm good to go. It's something you go to sleep with and you wake up with every day. It's not something that you can just be like "Hey, I'm going to take a day off here and I'll catch back up with it tomorrow." It's difficult to deal with. I think more than anything over the past three, four, five years is I've changed my diet a lot. I think that's made the biggest impact on me being able to control my numbers and being able to control diabetes.

I find it remarkable that this young man plays professional football with type 1 diabetes. I remember watching him wondering how his body was dealing with his injuries and fluctuations in his blood sugar levels due to the stressors of playing the game. Frankly, I don't know how he did it.

Celebrities with Type 2 Diabetes

Halle Berry (Academy Award–Winning Actress)[10]

Berry was in her early twenties when she became seriously ill and fell into a coma for one week. She was diagnosed with type 2 diabetes. Although her body was making some insulin, it wasn't enough to control her blood sugar levels. She needed insulin injections. Berry described her frightening situation.

One day, I simply passed out, and I didn't wake up for seven days, which is obviously very serious. They told me I might lose my eyesight, or I could lose my legs. I was scared to death, I thought I was going to die. I went into the hospital on my last breath, and came out feeling a hundred times better. I knew it was time to take better care of myself and I can honestly say that I am a healthier person than I was before I was taken ill...I feel very lucky that I can take insulin. It saves me from becoming ill. Diabetes turned out to be a gift. It gave me strength and toughness because I had to face reality, no matter how uncomfortable or painful it was.

She is a spokesman for the pharmaceutical company Novo Nordisk that makes products to help people live with their diabetes.

Tom Hanks (Academy Award–Winning Actor)[11]

Hanks shocked a David Letterman audience when he announced that he was diagnosed with type 2 diabetes at fifty-seven years old.

I went to the doctor and he said, "You know those high blood sugar numbers you've been dealing with since you were 36, well you've graduated. You've got type 2 diabetes, young man." Type 1 diabetes is very bad. Type 2 diabetes is controllable. You've got to lose weight and exercise a lot and change everything you eat...Sometimes I'm in pretty good shape, other times I'm not...it turns out, I do want to live.

Paula Deen (Daytime Emmy Award–Winner, Chef)[12]

Deen is a celebrated cook who had her own television show called *Paula's Best Dishes* and the author of numerous cookbooks. Her Southern specialties were generally deep fried, high in harmful saturated fats, and loaded with salt, sugar, and butter. She promoted harmful foods to millions of viewers. When asked about her unhealthy recipes, she told Oprah Winfrey, "Honey, I'm your cook, not your doctor. You have to be responsible for yourself."

She was diagnosed with type 2 diabetes three years before announcing that she had the disease. Deen has been criticized for promoting her unhealthy recipes to a hungry public while she knew of the potential risk for developing the disease. She modified her position and now encourages her fans to eat harmful foods in moderation.

The underlying question remains, did unhealthy eating cause her diabetes? Dr. Michael Dansinger of the Division of Endocrinology, Diabetes and Metabolism at Tufts Medical Center stated:

> It's an oversimplification to say that her cooking brought about her diabetes. Certainly eating high-fat and sugary foods leads to high caloric intake, which leads to obesity. But it's the obesity that increases the risk of developing type 2 diabetes. And obesity alone doesn't necessarily lead to the disease. Other risk factors, including genetic vulnerabilities, and an unhealthy, sedentary lifestyle, also raise the risk of diabetes. All of those stack the deck. And if you have the perfect storm of everything together, you may go on to develop diabetes.

Deen says she walks on a treadmill daily, has reduced her sweet tea habit, and is working on healthier versions of her famous recipes. Her son Bobby has a show called *Not My Mama's Meals* where he makes healthier recipes. She is making lifestyle changes and her current attitude is "I was determined to share my positive approach and not let diabetes stand in the way of enjoying my life."

Takeaway Points

Diabetes is a very scary and dangerous disease. Unfortunately, type 1 diabetes is not avoidable; however, there is a great deal that you can do to prevent type 2 diabetes. Healthier eating, increased physical activity, and weight management are the keys to preventing the disease. If you have diabetes, your lifestyle habits play a vital role in managing your elevated blood sugars. Learn about the disease and work closely with your healthcare provider to prevent serious complications such as a heart attack or stroke and you may live a longer, healthier, improved quality of life.

Additional Information

American Diabetes Association http://www.diabetes.org/

National Heart Lung and Blood Institute (NHLBI) (Protect Your Heart Against Diabetes) http://www.nhlbi.nih.gov/health/resources/heart/latino-diabetes-html

American Heart Association (Diabetes) http://www.heart.org/idc/groups/heart-public/@wcm/@hcm/documents/downloadable/ucm_300311.pdf.

The best diet is the one you don't know you're on.

—Psychologist, Brian Wansink

6

The Battle of the Bulge

The battle of the bulge is certainly a perfect title for this chapter. The statistics are startling. Nearly 70 percent of all American adults are either overweight or obese.[1] Most people who lose weight will regain it within five years.[2] If you are like the majority of Americans, you have struggled with maintaining a healthy weight for many years. You have probably tried a variety of strategies and diets to lose weight to no avail. The weight gain returns and you are getting discouraged. Your healthcare provider has warned you that you are at risk for diabetes or a heart attack, but you do not know how to begin or even what to do to keep the weight off. You may be wondering, "Does anything work?" "Why can't I lose this extra weight?"

I begin this chapter with information on the health complications of excess weight and the benefits of making even small changes in your life. You will learn how to identify your weight category. I also describe the unconscious triggers that cause overeating and review the latest research about food cravings. The chapter ends with a discussion of the common mistakes people make with weight loss and simple strategies that you may choose to incorporate into your daily life.

The Danger from Excess Weight

As we begin this section, I would like you to close your eyes and picture yourself carrying a bowling ball. It's heavy. Your arms hurt and you can't hold it for very long. If you dropped it on your foot, you would have a serious injury. In reality, a bowling ball weighs between six and sixteen pounds.[3] For women, think back to your last month of pregnancy. Most women gain at least thirty extra pounds. Remember your exhaustion, fatigue, and shortness of breath. Now think about the excess weight that you are carrying now. How many bowling balls or babies are you carrying around?

Your body is being traumatized by the constant pounding of all of that weight. The weight is taking its toll on all of the organs throughout your body. Everything is under a great deal of stress and strain. You don't feel well either. You are short of breath, your joints hurt, and you probably stopped looking in the mirror because you are tired of feeling bad. Your partner may be upset with you because that excess fat is blocking your airways and the snoring is keeping him or her up at night. That fat is intertwined within all of the organs of the body.

You are beginning to see the ramifications of this problem but feel so overwhelmed that you just do not know where to start to change it. As your weight increases, so does the extent of damage and additional complications.

Complications from Excess Weight[4]

Type 2 diabetes	Alzheimer's disease	Kidney stones
High blood pressure	Asthma	Fatty liver disease
Abnormal cholesterol	Cancer: many types	Kidney disease
Inflammation	Erectile dysfunction	Arthritis
Clotting disorders	Fertility problems	Surgical complications
Heart failure	Pregnancy complications	Nerve problems
Heart attack	Gall bladder disease	Gastric reflux disease
Stroke	Stomach discomforts	Gout
Blood clots to lower legs	Sleep apnea	Premature death
	Other Problems	
Absenteeism from work	Physical disability	Increased healthcare costs
Impaired quality of life	Aggressive behaviors	Depression/Low self esteem

*AHA Scientific Statement Population-Based Prevention of Obesity

Recognizing the harm of excess weight is an important first step. I've long argued that without this realization, why would a rational person change a lifestyle he or she loves. The bad news is that this list is a very long one. However, the good news is that it doesn't take many pounds to make a difference. Just losing 3 percent to 5 percent of your weight leads to clinical improvements in your health.[5] Don't get discouraged. I will show you the way out of this abyss, so hang in there with me a bit longer.

Weight Categories

You are probably wondering, "How bad is my weight problem?" There are two methods of weight measurement that were recommended in the latest obesity guidelines: body mass index (BMI) and waist circumference. For a copy of the guidelines, you may visit http://content.onlinejacc.org/article. aspx?articleid=1770219.

Body Mass Index (BMI)

The body mass index has been used for many years as a tool to describe healthy and unhealthy weight levels. The BMI is a calculation of your height and weight. The formula is:[6]

(weight in pounds) × 703 = BMI
(height in inches) squared

For example: The BMI for a 5'3" woman who weighs 200 pounds is 35.5.

200 pounds × 703 = BMI of 35.4245 or (rounded up) 35.5
63 inches × 63 inches

Once you have your BMI calculation, determine your weight classification. This woman has Class II obesity. The higher your BMI, the greater your risk for a heart attack and stroke.

Weight Classifications[6]

	BMI	Obesity Class
Underweight	<18.5	
Normal	18.5-24.9	
Overweight	25-29.9	
Obesity	30-34.9	Class I
Obesity	35-39.9	Class II
Extreme Obesity	≥40	Class III
*2013 Guidelines for the Management of Overweight and Obesity in Adults		

Another way to look at the BMI is within the tables in the appendix of this book. Find your height and weight. Move across the table. Your BMI may be found at the top. One criticism of relying on the BMI measurement for weight is that it is inaccurate in athletes. A football player who is fit may have a great deal of muscle which is heavier than fat. Let's say two men are each 6 feet tall and weigh 250 pounds. Their BMIs would be the same. However, one man is a Chicago Bear linebacker and the other a couch potato. The football player's weight has more muscle mass while the other man is mostly fat. In this case, the BMI is misleading. However, since most people are not as athletic as the linebacker, the BMI works well to calculate weight class.

Waist Circumference

Another way to calculate weight is to measure the waist circumference. Excess weight that is distributed around the waist represents abdominal fat. Think of abdominal fat as a living organ that releases substances harmful to the body, which increases risk for a heart attack. For women, the waist circumference should not exceed 35 inches, while for men, it should be less than 40 inches.[5] It is important to obtain an accurate measurement. Place the measuring tape at the level of the top or crest of the hipbone. Bring it straight across and record the number. The waist measurement of your pants may be different than your waist circumference.

Proper Waist Circumference Measurement[6]

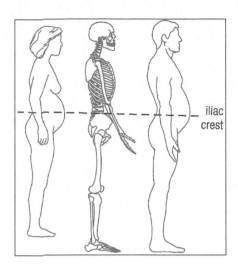

iliac
crest

The Practical Guide. Identification, Evaluation, and Treatment of Overweight and Obesity in Adults

National Heart, Lung, and Blood Institute; National Institutes of Health; US Department of Health and Human Services.

What is you BMI and waist circumference? Which weight category did you fall under? Take a moment and think about your weight. Are you in a danger zone? If you are in the Overweight, Obese Category I, II, or III, you fall into a danger zone. The higher category indicates greater health risks. Don't get discouraged. Recall that small losses of 3 percent to 5 percent of body weight will begin to improve your health.[5] Before I move into the simple strategies for you to consider, I want you to understand the psychology of overeating. I will describe some exciting research conducted by psychologist Brian Wansink. His work is revolutionizing how we think about overeating.

Psychology of Overeating

Psychologists have contributed a great deal to our understanding of those unconscious influences that sabotage the best intentions to lose weight. I believe that this is the secret weapon to gaining control of your weight problem. You must understand how you are unconsciously interfering with your weight loss. The truth is that we are all vulnerable to unconscious influences to overeat, no matter our waist size.

Brian Wansink is currently the Cornell University Food and Brand Lab director. In 2007, he was appointed by the White House as the USDA executive director in charge of the Food Pyramid and dietary guidelines. His research became so influential that he is responsible for the 100 calorie individual servings that are now available on grocery store shelves. His work has been presented on various television shows as well. I highly recommend his books, *Mindless Eating: Why We Eat More Than We Think* and *Slim By Design: Mindless Eating Solutions for Everyday Life*. You can also view a short YouTube presentation titled: "Professor Brian Wansink on Why We Eat More Than We Need" by visiting https://www.youtube.com/watch?v=8Ogsmh_czeY. The following section highlights some of his work and will raise your awareness of common mistakes people make who overeat and the simple strategies that can be implemented to lose weight.

Stale Movie Popcorn[7]

During a matinee, 161 moviegoers who were full from eating lunch were given a free coupon for a soft drink and popcorn. They randomly received either a large or medium container of stale popcorn that was five days old. One participant described the popcorn, "It was like Styrofoam packing peanuts (17)."[8] Upon leaving the theatre, the containers were weighed and the participants completed a brief survey. Results showed that the participants that liked the popcorn ate 49 percent more if they were given the larger container compared to those who received the medium container. Interestingly, those who did not like the popcorn ate 61 percent more if given the larger container compared to the medium container. Wansink believes that people mindlessly eat more from larger containers.

Ice Cream Social[9]

Following an event, 85 portion control nutritional experts were invited to an ice cream social. The participants were divided into four groups and given a:

- Large scoop with a large bowl
- Large scoop with a small bowl
- Small scoop with a large bowl
- Small scoop with a small bowl

They served themselves ice cream. While the participants completed a brief survey, the bowl of ice cream was weighed.

The people given the larger bowl served themselves and ate 31 percent more ice cream than those given a smaller bowl. If they also had a larger scoop, they ate 57 percent more than those given the smaller bowl and scoop. These highly educated nutritionists were fooled by the larger utensils. Wansink stated:

> People tend to eat 92 percent of the food that they serve to themselves…obese patients may want to use smaller bowls and spoons…to feel less like they are 'sacrificing' or 'on a diet'. (243)

Wine Connoisseurs[10]

At Wansink's food laboratory/restaurant, 49 participants were given the same meal along with a glass of $2 Charles Shaw cabernet wine also known as Two Buck Chuck. The wine was relabeled "New from Noah's Winery in California" and "New from Noah's Winery in North Dakota." The group that drank the California brand said that they enjoyed their meal more, took longer to eat, and ate 12 percent more food compared to the North Dakota wine group. Although the wine was exactly the same, participants ate more food when drinking from what they perceived was a higher quality wine.

The Bottomless Soup Bowl[11]

A table was configured so that participants could eat soup from an 18-ounce bowl that continuously refilled when half of the soup had been consumed. They were unaware that the bowl kept refilling to remain half full. The other participants were given an 18-ounce bowl that did not refill. All 54 participants were allowed to eat the soup for 20 minutes. A brief questionnaire was completed at the end of the session and the soup measured. The group that did not get the visual cues that the bowl was emptying ingested 73 percent more soup than the group whose bowl emptied. Wansink thought that the people who saw their soup bowl emptying slowed their eating and ate less because of the visual cues. The bowl is emptying and it is time to stop eating.

Super Bowl Chicken Wing Party[12]

Wansink invited 50 graduate students (recently taught about portion control) to a Super Bowl party at a sports bar and served chicken wings. The waitresses were to remove the bones from half of the tables. The participants that were allowed to see the bones pile up ate 28 percent less chicken wings than those whose bones were immediately removed. Evidence of the bones piled up seemed to moderate eating behavior.

M&M's Color Temptation[13]

Everyone knows that M&M's candies taste exactly the same no matter the color coatings. Wansink invited 105 adults to view a video and served M&M's. Half of the participants were given a bowl with 7 different M&M's colors while the other participants received a bowl with 10 different M&M's colors. The bowls were removed and weighed while the participants completed a brief survey. The group that ate from the bowl with 10 different colors ate on average 77 percent more M&M's and said that they "had more fun." Wansink stated:[8]

> The first bite of anything is almost always the best. The second a little less, the third less again. At some point, we're tired of the yogurt or cake. But if we add two more types of yogurt, or if we add ice cream to the cake, our taste buds are back to the races. (72)

The participants had to keep trying all of the colors. This explains why buffets and parties with a variety of food choices are dangerous environments for weight loss. Without even realizing it, people want to try everything.

Hershey Kisses Temptation[14]

A candy bowl of chocolate Hershey Kisses was placed on the desk of 16 secretaries. For 3 weeks, they received one of three options:

- Candy bowl placed on the top of their desk.
- Candy bowl placed inside their drawer.
- Candy bowl placed several few feet away.

Each night, the candy was counted and the bowls refilled. At the end of the week, the bowls were rotated so that each secretary eventually received all three options. Each week, a brief survey was completed. Wansink wrote:[8]

> The typical secretary ate about nine chocolates a day if they were sitting on her desk staring right at her. That's about 225 extra calories a day. If she had to go to the effort of opening the desk drawer, she did so only six times a day. If she had to get up and walk six feet to get a chocolate, she ate only four…When we talked to the secretaries after the study, many of them mentioned that having six feet between them and the candy gave them enough time to think twice whether they really wanted it. It gave them time to talk themselves out of having another chocolate. (85)

The pause gave them a few seconds to decide not to eat it. The craving passed. Food cravings are somewhat like a contraction during childbirth. It takes a few minutes to peak and then it subsides. Making it a little harder to satisfy the craving may allow you to decide that you don't really want it after all.

I noticed over the years that my friends and coworkers who struggle with weight often keep chocolates or other candies at their desk. A good simple strategy is to keep it out of sight or remove it altogether. If you have to get up to go to the vending machine to eat that chocolate, the time and effort may dissuade you from doing it. The opposite approach also works with healthy foods. Keep them easily and readily available.

Comfort Foods for Men and Women[8]

Finally, Wansink gave 1,004 American adults a long list of comfort foods and asked them to check off their favorites. He found large differences between men and women. The foods rated highly by women were "ice cream, chocolate and cookies" while the men preferred "ice cream, soup, pizza, or pasta (141)." The men also rated "hot foods" and "meal-like food" higher than women. Men said that these foods made them feel "spoiled," "pampered," "taken care of," or "waited on," while women felt those foods reminded them of the work required to prepare it. Women preferred quick snack foods that were "hassle-free." It makes the point that when trying to lose weight, men and women may have very different vulnerabilities and temptations.

Illusion of Size

Take a look at the following diagram. Which center dot looks bigger to you?

The Dot Test[15]

*Adapted from Ebbinghaus-Tichener size contrast illusion.

They are the same size. Did you get it right? Your mind may have monetarily tricked you to see the center dot surrounded by the smaller dots as bigger. The point to this exercise is that you can use this optical illusion with food as well. Placing your food on a smaller plate may appear like you are eating a larger portion of food. Wansink recommends this strategy for weight loss as you will feel more satisfied, eat less, and lose weight.[8]

After reading this section I hope that you are more aware that overeating is a problem that occurs in our unconscious as well as within our conscious choices. Wansink's new book, *Slim by Design* helps the reader understand the environmental changes that set you up for greater weight loss success.

Depression/Negative Mood States

Depression, anxiety, stress, and other negative mood states interfere with weight loss. I believe that chronic negative mood states must be treated before serious weight loss can occur. Not all people who struggle with weight are depressed, but many use eating to lift a negative mood.[16] Endorphins are "feel good" chemicals in the brain. They increase with food, exercise, a variety of pleasurable activities, smoking, and drugs. New research is examining whether people who struggle with excess weight were born with low levels of endorphins.[17] People may overeat to increase the "feel good" chemicals, but it only works momentarily. In my experience, many people are embarrassed to admit this problem. They suffer for years, accumulating weight and harmful health consequences. I recommend that if you think that you may be suffering from depression, speak with your healthcare provider about a treatment plan that best fits your needs.

The Danger of Boredom

Boredom is another common trigger for mindless eating. It's a huge problem. Stop for a moment and think about the activities that you love. For some of you, it may be gardening, for others sports, for still others quilting. Can you get a part-time job doing it or can you volunteer in this area? If you love to bike in the mountains, can you get a job in a bike store? If you love working with children, can you volunteer at your local school to help children learn to read? Finding fulfilling things to do keeps you busy and helps prevent overeating.

Thus far, I spent a great deal of time focusing on the psychological issues related to overeating. In the next section, I will get into the importance of portion control and specific strategies that you may consider to help with weight management.

Portion Control

Portion sizes have changed dramatically within the past thirty years and correlate with the obesity epidemic. A study conducted by the Center for Disease Control (CDC) and Prevention examined American food consumption between 1971 and 2000.[18] During this time period, obesity rates doubled. The researchers found that caloric intake increased in women from 1,542 calories on average a day to 1,877 and men increased from 2,450 calories a day to 2,618. They surmised that the increase in caloric intake and waistlines was most likely due to the decision of the restaurant industry to increase portion sizes two to five times bigger than in previous generations. Dr. Gary Foster, of the Weight and Eating Disorders Program at the University of Pennsylvania School of Medicine stated:

> We've become more overweight as a country as candy bars are now king-sized and sodas are supersized. It's much tougher to manage your weight in this environment than it was in 1970. (2)

The typical hamburger meal, purchased by adults in the 1960s, was comparable to a children's meal today: a small cheeseburger, a small fry, and today's kid-size Coke (12 ounces). The entire meal contained around 500 calories.[19] Fast forward to today and everything has been super-sized. Most adult Americans typically order a much larger burger, a large fry, and a large Coke (30 ounces), weighing in at a whopping 1,300 to 1,600 calories.[19] No wonder we have such an obesity problem across the nation. We have lost our sense of what a normal portion should be. We think that whatever is placed in front of us is the amount that we are supposed to eat. In order to regain control of your weight, you need to start thinking differently about what constitutes an appropriate portion.

Portion Label

A good way to start understanding an appropriate portion size is to read the package label. I will return to the ice cream label from chapter 3 to make this point.

Brand A and Brand B Saturated Fat Food Label

Chocolate Ice Cream Brand A		Chocolate Ice Cream Brand B	
Serving size	½ cup	Serving size	½ cup
Calories per serving	260	Calories per serving	100
Total fat	17(g)	Total fat	3.5(g)
Saturated fat	10(g)	Saturated fat	2(g)
Trans fat	0.5(g)	Trans fat	0(g)
Cholesterol	90(mg)	Cholesterol	15(mg)
Sodium	45(mg)	Sodium	30(mg)
Total carbohydrates	22(g)	Total carbohydrates	15(g)
Dietary fiber	0(g)	Dietary fiber	1(g)
Sugars	19(g)	Sugars	13(g)
Protein	5(g)	Protein	3(g)

You can see that a portion is ½ cup of ice cream. I doubt many of us stick with just ½ cup. Recall that we have to adjust the label content based upon what we are actually eating. As you look at the labels, you can see that Brand B has fewer calories than

Brand A. It might be worth trying Brand B. After some time, you probably may not notice the difference in flavor but would cut more than half of the calories.

Compare the amount of food that you eat regularly with these established portion sizes.

Single Serving or Portion Size[20]

Grain Products	Vegetables and Fruits
1 cup of cereal = fist	1 cup of salad greens = baseball
1 pancake = CD	1 baked potato = fist
½ cup cooked rice, pasta, potato = 1/2 baseball	1 medium fruit = baseball
	½ cup fresh fruit = 1/2 baseball
1 slice of bread = cassette tape	¼ cup raisins = 1 large egg
1 peace cornbread = bar of soap	
Dairy and Cheese	**Meat and Alternatives**
1 ½ oz. cheese = 4 stacked dice or 2 cheese slices	3 oz meat, fish and poultry = deck of cards
½ cup of ice cream = ½ baseball	3 oz grilled/baked fish = checkbook
	2 Tablespoons peanut butter = ping pong ball
Fats	
1 teaspoon margarine or spreads = 1 dice	
* Portion Control Preventive Cardiovascular Nurses Association (PCNA)	

Daily Portions

The Food Pyramid was developed by the government to help the public consume a healthy diet. While Americans continued to gain weight, the Food Pyramid was too confusing for most people, and a newer approach was needed. Government nutrition experts developed the Choose My Healthy Plate program in the hopes that it would be easier to follow and reduce obesity. You may visit www.choosemyplate.gov to view both plans. Use the Food Pyramid or Choose My Plate model to give you a better idea of healthy daily portions.

Comparison between My Food Pyramid and Choose My Plate[21]

	Grains	Fresh Fruits and Vegetables	Milk	Meat & Beans
Food Pyramid	Eat 6 ounces of whole grains/day 1 oz=1 slice bread, 1 cup cereal, ½ cup cooked rice	Eat 2 1/2 cups of vegetables a day Eat 2 cups of fresh fruits a day Avoid juices	Drink 3 cups low fat /day	Eat 5 1/2 ounces lean meats/day
Healthy Plate	Fill your plate with 1/4 whole grains	1/4 of your plate in vegetables 1/4 of your plate in fresh fruits	8 oz. low-fat milk or water with each meal	1/4 of your plate with lean meats
*Adapted from www.choosemyplate.gov				

Diagram of My Food Pyramid and Choose My Plate[21]

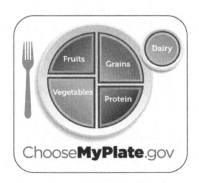

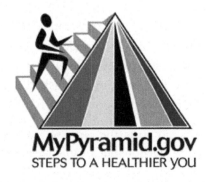

Both systems encourage exercise and reducing harmful fats, and sweets. It comes down to a balance between the calories consumed versus the calories burned. If you ingest more calories than you burn, you will gain weight. If you burn more calories than you ingest, you will lose weight. The recommended caloric intake for weight loss is between 1,200 to 1,500 calories a day for women and 1,500 to 1,800 calories a day for men.[5] Take a moment to think about how much you are eating each day. Look at the label on some of your common foods. You may be shocked where you are getting the extra calories. Try substituting healthier lower calorie choices wherever you can.

The Restaurant Industry

I'm a big fan of restaurants having the freedom to offer whatever products they think are best to sell to their consumers. However, I appreciate it when restaurants offer healthier options as well. Try to find items with lower salt, less saturated fat and sugar, and smaller portions. Unfortunately, those options are few and far between.

Personal Story

I was a cardiac nurse educator teaching courses on cholesterol, blood pressure, and portion control at a heart institute near Chicago. The cafeteria of this prestigious institution only sold food in very large portions. One day, I decided to visit the manager to inquire why smaller portion options were not available for purchase. This event occurred in 2006 when the dangers of obesity were widely known. I asked the manager if he would consider selling smaller portions. He told me:

> It costs the same to make a larger portion as a smaller portion, but I can charge a great deal more for the larger

size. I can't cut back on the size. I would lose money and
my director would be unhappy with me.

His attitude explains the huge portion problem throughout
the restaurant food industry. It comes down to profit. Most
restaurant food is loaded with salt, sugar, and saturated fat, and
the portions are large enough to feed three people. No wonder we
have an obesity problem.

Just be aware that whenever you eat out, it may not be good for
your blood pressure, cholesterol, or waistline. Consider ordering
from the kids' menu. You will be surprised how full you will feel.
Thirty years ago, these were the correct portion sizes for adults.
Share an adult entree or only eat half and save the rest for another
meal. My husband and I often share an entree and order an extra
side salad. This practice also saves money.

Another great idea is to order a side salad and ask for grilled
chicken to be placed on top of it. Consider adding lean meat to
the side salad rather than eating it alone. Selecting fish when you
eat out is a great time to get your healthy omega fats. Salmon is
a great choice. Be careful of the bread placed on your table and
avoid the extra appetizer and dessert. The entree should be more
than enough food. If you must have it, pick one but not both:
appetizer or dessert and share it. If you do run into that rare
restaurant that offers a healthier alternative, please compliment
the owner. We need to reinforce good behavior whenever we see
it. Slow down and enjoy your meal.

Bon Appetit!

Frequency of Eating to Reduce Food Cravings

In the previous sections, you learned about the unconscious
influences of overeating and proper portion size. In this section,
I will address the frequency of eating to stabilize blood sugar.
When I speak in front of groups, I always ask this one question.

Rarely does anyone get it right. What do you think is the single *biggest* mistake that people make who struggle with excess weight? Take a minute and ponder the question. In my opinion, the single *biggest* mistake that people make who are trying to lose weight but keep failing is that they "skip meals." The meal almost universally skipped is breakfast.

Importance of Breakfast

Breakfast means "to break the fast." You have been sleeping all night in a fasting state. Because you are sleeping and not eating, the liver secretes a small amount of glucose or sugar throughout the night for energy that the organs need. Going from a sleeping state to wakefulness is very stressful on your body. Your body needs blood sugar to get going and face the day. It's looking for food.

Let's say that you eat a pure carbohydrate for breakfast such as a bowl of sweetened cereal. Your body will break that food down immediately and convert it to glucose or blood sugar. The pancreas senses that sugar floating in the blood and wants to help drive it into the cells to combine with oxygen to make energy. It releases a great deal of insulin. Recall that insulin is the hormone that moves the sugar into the cell where it will be used. The blood sugar is quickly used up by the body. The good news is that your brain and body loved the food that you just ate. Your metabolism is revved up and you are energized to face the day. The bad news is that your pancreas excreted a large amount of insulin. Because of the extra insulin, the sugar in the blood is no longer available. This leads to symptoms from low blood sugar, which may include: jittery, shaky, irritable, hunger, etc. You may be thinking, "I would have been better off not eating. If I don't eat anything, I can go all day without feeling hungry. It's only been two hours and I'm hungry again." It is at this point where most people misunderstand what is happening to their physiology. The food that you ate turned on your metabolism. You are burning calories and gearing up to take on the day. If you are trying to lose weight, burning calories any way you can is the goal! Hunger is not a bad thing. What your body is telling you, "I like what you sent me…send me some more food."

The problem with eating a breakfast high in carbohydrates without protein is that your body will burn through that food very quickly and cause low blood sugar symptoms. A smarter plan is to eat a single piece of toast with peanut butter. The fat and the protein in the peanut butter take longer to breakdown. The sugar enters your blood more slowly. You may be hungry again within two hours, but you shouldn't experience the low blood sugar symptoms. An egg with a piece of toast works too. When I'm on the run, I like to eat a lower calorie protein bar for a quick breakfast with my coffee. The protein in the nuts sticks with me. Oatmeal is another great choice. The key concept here is to recognize that your body needed the food that you sent it, and two hours later, it is asking for more. Embrace what your body needs. Feed it again. Plan for this situation. Eat a piece of fruit or ¼ cup or a handful of trail mix. Be sure the trail mix contains some type of nuts for added protein. Your blood sugar will be stabilized. For weight loss, you need to keep your metabolism revved up all day. I recommend three small meals and three small snacks. Include a bit of protein with each one, but remember to watch those portion sizes and keep an eye on your caloric intake. You will begin to feel better as you are getting the nutrition that your body needs and you should start shedding pounds.

Binge Eating

What happens when you skip breakfast or other meals? In the short term, you may feel like this is healthy; however, it causes long-term problems. Your body will get the sugar it needs, no matter what, so it will begin breaking down muscle and fat for energy. In the process, fatty acids or ketones are left behind. Your blood becomes more acidic and you often lose your appetite. Some people may experience a tiny bit of nausea. For someone trying to lose weight, they may be misled into thinking that the loss of appetite is a good thing. It is not. When you skip meals, your brain thinks that you are starving. It shuts your entire body down, preserving your fat and calories for future needs. This in effect slows down metabolism and makes weight loss very difficult. Your brain doesn't know if you are just skipping a meal or headed off for the television show *Survivor*. In the "starvation mode," your brain is holding on to fat for dear life. If you do this often, the brain begins to lose trust in you to send it regular meals and remains in starvation mode. Losing weight becomes even more difficult. You think that you are being so smart to control your hunger, but in reality, your body is refusing to lose weight. This situation is the exact opposite of what you want to accomplish.

You can remain in this starvation mode until about 2:00 p.m. At that point your brain overrides the best of your intentions and literally starts screaming for food. You can't shovel it in fast enough and you are now binging! In addition, it is very hard on your organs to digest all of that food in one setting. The best approach for weight loss is to eat the right foods more frequently. Don't ignore hunger. Feed your body, but be smart about it. I recommend that you eat something small for breakfast every day. Add a small snack two hours later as your blood sugar drops and you experience hunger. Eat an appropriate lunch and again be ready for a small snack when your feel hungry two hours later. Enjoy an appropriate dinner and another light snack two hours later if you are hungry. A good rule of thumb is to keep your snacks around 100 calories.

Liquid Food

As you are selecting healthy foods, I highly recommend that you *avoid* liquid snacks and meals. The goal is to help stabilize your blood sugar levels. Liquids of any kind are digested rapidly. You can drink a great deal of calories very quickly. Liquid food fools the brain. Although you may have consumed a great deal of calories, the brain doesn't sense it as with solid food, which makes you feel fuller for two reasons. First, the food stretches the stomach bands and sends a message to your brain that you are full. Secondly, the food takes longer to digest and enters your blood sugar more slowly. Consuming drinks such as smoothies does not require the digestive system to break down the food. The blender did all of the work. The higher the fiber content of the food, the longer it takes to break the food down, and you burn more calories.

Avoid liquids such as fruit juices and smoothies whenever you can. Eat the solid food instead. If you are someone who loves smoothies, keep your portion to less than 8 ounces. Persons with diabetes are not allowed to drink fruit juices because they are rapidly digested and enter the blood quickly as sugar or glucose. Sweetened sodas are a major problem for people trying to lose weight. Try carbonated flavored seltzer water or sparkling water instead. Place a lime, orange, or lemon wedge in a glass of ice water. I think you will be surprised how refreshing the water will be. It will hydrate you without all of the calories. I will address artificial sweeteners later in this chapter. I recommend that you restrict artificial drinks to less than one a day and avoid all regular soft drinks as much as possible. If you have to have a soda, grab the smaller 8-ounce size.

Dining

There are many things that you can consider during mealtimes to promote weight loss. I will provide some suggestions for each meal.

Breakfast

I've already described some creative options for you. The idea is to eat something. Be sure it contains some amount of protein. If you aren't used to eating breakfast, try a protein bar, but watch the calories. Some of them are loaded. Try to keep it under 200 calories. A single piece of peanut butter toast is another quick idea, but be careful to keep the amount of peanut butter under one or two tablespoons. Eating something gets your metabolism started.

Lunch

Pack a lunch if you can. If you eat out for lunch, eat half of the sandwich that you order and save the other half or split it with a coworker who is also trying to lose weight. You can also order a small side salad and ask for grilled chicken to be placed on top. If you have to order a large entrée-sized salad remember it is meant for two or three people, so take much of it home. A kids' meal may be a great idea for lunch as well.

Dinner

Home-cooked dinners are best but not always feasible. My Crock-Pot has become my best friend. You can place any meat with any can of soup and let it cook all day on low. You can also throw in vegetables and dinner will be ready when you get home. Experiment with different meats and soup flavors. If you have high blood pressure, it may be better to remove half of the soup from the can and fill the remaining can with water to lower the salt content. Fill your plate with an array of colorful vegetables. Uncooked vegetables provide more nutrient value than cooked vegetables and are harder to digest, which burns more calories. Steaming them is a low-calorie option as well. Your meat serving should be about the size of a deck of cards. Have fun and enjoy your meals.

Snacks

Regular snacks throughout the day are a great way to keep your metabolism going. Always keep an eye on the amount that you are eating and calorie content. A piece of fruit, a palm size of nuts, or ¼ cup of any type of trail mix are good options.

Dessert

Life is meant to be enjoyed and food is a wonderful part of life. Eat your meal and wait twenty minutes before you eat your dessert. Keep it small and experiment with healthier options. It can be difficult to make them healthy, but it can be done. For those of you who are like me and have a terrible sweet tooth, don't deny yourself. Thanks to Wansink's research, there are many 100 calorie items now available on your grocery store shelf. If you need to bake cookies, add raisins, nuts, and oatmeal using less sugar. A woman that I interviewed for this book is a wonderful baker who has kept her weight off for many years. She told me that she bakes a dessert for an event but never brings it home. Finally, I make a great cake that we call the Julie Cake after my deceased sister-in-law who was an amazing baker as well. I only make desserts such as this one for special occasions. If I have it around all the time, I will eat it!

Julie Cake

Bake a dark chocolate cake mix as directed in 2 round pans. Cool for 15 minutes and then remove from the pans. When completely cooled, place in the freezer for 30 minutes. Remove from the freezer and slice each layer into 2 (round) halves. Add low-fat, low-calorie cool whip between each layer. When finished, frost with dark chocolate fudge frosting. You can also experiment with other flavors. It looks rich but is really a great alternative and a wonderful dessert. Serve yourself a small piece for special occasions.

Dangerous Pitfalls

One of the beautiful things about life are the celebrations that bring so much joy. However, they can be dangerous pitfalls for people struggling to maintain a healthy weight. One of my obese patients was a young woman who was eating healthier foods, feeling better, and beginning to shed pounds. She was concerned about relapse during an upcoming wedding. We worked on a strategy that really helped her get through the event. She danced, had fun, and enjoyed the wonderful food but ate only small portions of it. She decided to be good the day before and the day after the wedding. She told me she had a great time and it worked. She didn't binge eat nor did she feel like she was on a diet.

Recently, I made my husband his favorite birthday meal of turkey with gravy, mashed potatoes, broccoli with cheese, dressing, a lemon cake, and served white wine with dinner. This type of meal had the potential to sabotage any weight loss plan, not to mention blood pressure and cholesterol control. I took my own advice and enjoyed all of it but in very small portions. The bottom line is to enjoy life. Food is a major component of many of our celebrations. Don't deny yourself that joy but be sensible about it and never eat to the point of feeling stuffed like my turkey.

Healthy Eating through the Holidays

The holidays are a vulnerable time. Generally, the foods are high in calories, butter, sugar, and fat so be careful. Enjoy them, but be sensible. There are a few options that other patients have found helpful. Eat a full meal before you go to the party. If you go with a full stomach, you will tend to graze less. Try the foods but only small bites or portions. If you are bringing an item, make it fun but heart healthy. A vegetable tray with a flavorful dip is always a good choice. My friends and family love my garden salad. I literally toss a variety of colorful vegetables into it and serve a homemade Italian dressing made with olive oil or a low fat buttermilk ranch dressing. If you are attending a party, eat healthy the day before and the day after the event. Exercise the day of the party. Do something to make up for the extra caloric content that you might consume. Have fun and don't deprive yourself of a good time. Just be sensible and you can "have your cake and eat it too."

Daily Weights

According to the latest guidelines, it is recommended that you weigh yourself frequently.[5] The thinking is that if you begin to gain weight you will be motivated to adjust your lifestyle to keep it in check. Research has indicated that those who weigh themselves frequently manage their weight more effectively.[2] I weigh myself daily, and if weight starts to creep up, I stop and think, "Did I eat a lot of salt or was it extra junk food?" Sometimes, you will just have a terrible craving for something or a bad day and your weight may climb. Weighing yourself frequently helps you make a correction if your weight starts to climb again.

Exercise

The latest guidelines recommend that you engage in aerobic activity for thirty minutes a day on most days of the week.[5] For weight loss, forty minutes a day is recommended.[5] Of course, this advice is great, but only 20 percent of people will actually do it.[22] This recommendation is not realistic for most people. If you are a couch potato and you know who you are, start slow. There are a few more realistic alternatives for you to consider. Go for a five- or ten-minute walk with a loved one. It's a great stress buster. Walk five minutes from your house and then come back. If you do that three times a day, you just met the exercise requirements. Fill your life with active things that you love to do. For weight loss, a little bit of weight training goes a very long way. Muscle is heavier than fat and metabolically burns more calories compared to stored fat. However, get a physical and talk with your healthcare provider before you start a serious exercise program. The key is to be as active as possible and "all" activity counts. In chapter 8, I describe exercise in more detail. For now, just realize that the more active you are, the more calories you will burn.

Halo Effect

Wansink described the Halo Effect as the tendency to view a food as healthy, and therefore, you can eat more of it because it is good for you.[8] Foods labeled "sugar free" and "low fat" are especially problematic. Often, when the fat content is reduced, the sugar content goes up, and the overall caloric content remains unchanged. The reverse is also true for sugar content. When sugar content is lowered, fat content goes up and calories often remain unchanged. You think that you are eating the healthier item, but in reality, you are still consuming a great deal of calories because you are eating too much. Take a look at the following label.

Comparison of One Serving of Chocolate Cake

	Sugar Free Mix	Regular Mix	Major Restaurant
Calories	310	370	1,000 to 1,600
Saturated Fat	3	2.5	26
Transfat	1.5	1.5	NA
Sodium	350	415	1,430

First, you will note that there isn't much difference between the sugar-free cake label and the regular cake label. Yet I think that many of us get fooled into thinking "sugar free" means no calories so we may tend to eat more. The real shock comes from the restaurant chocolate cake. It's luxurious but loaded with many more calories, fat, and salt. In fact, one serving is more than an entire day's worth of saturated fat that is recommended for most people. Just be careful when you see "sugar free" or "low fat." Finally, some people fall prey to the "halo effect" when it comes to exercise as well. "I exercised today, therefore I can eat more food." Keep an eye on the number of calories and serving sizes that you are consuming. A calorie is a calorie and too many leads to increased weight.

Popular Diets

Any "diet" will work in the short term to help you lose weight. Some are more restrictive than others. Whenever you reduce your calories or increase your physical activity, you will lose weight. The real questions are: "How much weight can I lose?" How fast will I lose it?" "Can I keep it off?" I'm not a fan of any diet and have used the phrase, "Diet is a four-letter word." It feels too restrictive to me. I like to think in terms of realistic choices and setting the environment up for success. However, some people like more structure. In this section, I provide you with information on some of the more popular diets. I end with a comment on starvation diets and a summary of the recommendations that I suggest for patients. Personally, I find following diets too difficult to maintain, but each person must find the plan that works best for them.

The *US News and World Report* asked nutrition and weight loss experts across the nation to evaluate and rank twenty-seven popular diets. You may visit their Web site for additional information at: http://health.usnews.com/best-diet. The diets were evaluated on the ability to meet short- and long-term weight loss goals, ease to follow, nutrition quality, safety, diabetes and heart risk reductions. Points were awarded for positive aspects of the diet and tallied for an overall score.

Paleo Diet[23] (16.5 Out of 40 Possible Points)

The Paleo diet has become very popular in the past few years. The premise of the diet is to eat like our hunter-gatherer primitive ancestors from the Paleolithic period 10,000 years ago. If the caveman didn't eat it, you shouldn't eat it either. Prohibited foods are dairy products rich in calcium, whole grains high in fiber, vitamins and minerals, legumes high in protein, sugar, and processed foods.[24] There have been a few positive studies published in reputable journals, but they were extremely small studies and conducted for a very short time. Further, any time you restrict calories for any reason, you will lose weight. It is the weight loss that improves your blood pressure, blood sugar, and cholesterol. The real question is how does the diet impact your quality of life and can you sustain it over time? I support the idea of eating more vegetables, lean meats, and less processed foods, but I don't like the idea of banning certain foods. Eating food is part of the joy in life. I can't imagine life devoid of an occasional piece of "processed" cake or as Kurtis Hiatt said in the *US News and World Report* article: "Can you get used to the idea of breadless sandwiches? Or having your milk and cookies without either milk and cookies."

Atkins (19.5 Out of 40 Points)[23]

The Atkins diet is high in protein such as eggs, chicken, and meat and low in carbohydrates such as sugars, potatoes, white bread, and rice. Without carbohydrates, the body begins to burn fat and weight begins to drop. It takes longer to break down dietary protein and fat so you feel fuller longer. In addition, ketones are produced when fat is burned which causes a loss in appetite and further weight reductions. This diet sounds great except that the price for the weight loss may be too high. The ketones may damage the kidneys and LDL (bad) cholesterol levels may become too high. In recent years, the diet has promoted eating healthier dietary fat and avoiding saturated fats. If you are going to try this diet, work with your healthcare provider to ensure that your diet plan includes adequate nutrition, your LDL cholesterol is in check, and your kidneys are working properly. You may find that this eating plan is too challenging to follow and very difficult to sustain over time.

South Beach Diet (23.5 Out of 40 Points)[23]

I must confess that I am a huge fan of cardiologist Dr. Arthur Agatston who developed the South Beach Diet. He is a pioneer in the prevention of heart attack and stroke and developed the scale used to quantify the coronary artery calcium heart scan described in chapter 2. A few years ago, he noticed that his practice consisted of mostly overweight or obese patients. This observation led him to examine the connection between excess weight and cardiovascular disease. His journey led him to write his first book, but I recommend his more recent book titled *The South Beach Heart Program* to my patients.

The diet encourages the consumption of a great deal of vegetables, eggs, low-fat dairy, lean meats such as turkey and chicken, whole grains, and nuts. Foods to avoid are: bagels, white bread, potatoes, cookies, ice cream, honey, jam, pineapple, watermelon, and raisins, which are high in natural sugar. Following this diet helps to stabilize blood sugar in order to reduce food cravings. He also asks participants to exercise twenty minutes every day. While those recommendations are good, most obese people will find it too hard to stick to this plan. My patients have complained that the recipes are difficult to prepare. However, his books are excellent resources that help to explain foods that raise blood sugar levels and trigger cravings. This book also contains invaluable information on the process of heart disease.

Jenny Craig (29 Out of 40 Points)[23]

I'm not a big fan of prepackaged meals because I think they are more expensive than most people can afford. However, some of my patients love the structure of the prepared meals and lose weight. They are well balanced and range anywhere from 1,200 to 2,000 calories depending upon your activity level. You are sent three meals a day with two snacks and a dessert included with dinner. The portions are controlled for you. The cost varies from city to city but on average runs $100 a week with a one-time sign-on fee of $400. The major benefit of this plan is that you do not have to prepare your meals and there is no calorie or carbohydrate counting. You just eat the food sent to you. My concern about this diet is that when you stop the program, you will not know how to eat properly, and the weight will return.

Mediterranean Diet (29.5 Out of 40 Points)[23]

Researchers found that people living in the Mediterranean region have less heart disease and half the obesity levels as Americans.[25]

While each country may vary in their eating habits, generalities do exist. They tend to eat more fruits and vegetables, whole grains, beans, nuts, legumes, olive oil, fish, poultry, eggs, healthier cheese, and yogurt. Sweets and red meats are limited and a glass of red wine compliments their dinner. It is also well known that they eat smaller portions and live more active lives. There are a variety of options in foods, and this is a diet pattern that one can enjoy and sustain for the rest of your life. I like the lifestyle of the Mediterraneans. You may visit www.americanheart.org for more information on this diet.

Weight Watchers (30.5 Out of 40 Points)[23]

Weight Watchers is a diet plan that has been around for a long time and was recently updated to a newer point system. Foods are rated for their health and caloric content. You are limited to a certain amount of points each day. Fresh fruits and vegetables have 0 points and presumably you can eat as many as you like. You are encouraged to eat three meals a day with two snacks. The plan is simple whether you are at home or eating out. No food is denied, but portions are limited. The monthly program costs $39.95, individual weekly meetings are between $12 and $14 with a $20 sign on fee. I especially like this plan for people who carry fifty pounds or more of excess weight. You get to eat a larger quantity of the right types of food and do not feel hungry if you stick to the plan. If you have less than thirty pounds of excess weight, Weight Watchers may work for you, but a professional dietitian may be better suited to fine-tune your eating to help you lose those last pounds.

DASH Diet (31 Out of 40 Points)[23]

I described the Dietary Approach to Stopping Hypertension (DASH) diet in chapter 4. This diet encourages you to eat a variety of fruits and vegetables, low-fat dairy, lean meats, less salt, sweets, and processed foods. Many studies have supported that eating a diet rich in fruits and vegetables lowers blood pressure. Eating the DASH way will also improve your cholesterol, blood sugar, and promote weight loss. The DASH plan is a good choice and another great way to think about your eating. You can remain on it for the rest of your life.

Starvation Diets

I hope that I have made the point that starvation diets "never" work for sustained weight loss! You can lose the weight, but it will come right back once you start eating more food again. Binging is a huge potential problem. According to the latest obesity guidelines, you should never restrict your caloric intake to under 800 calories without the care of a physician.[5] Weight loss should be slow so that your body does not enter the "starvation mode." If you lose weight too fast, your metabolism may shut down and your body will hold on to fat. A one- to two-pound weight loss per week is ideal.[26] In regards to weight loss, you want to be the tortoise, not the hare.

Living for a Healthy Heart Plan

I like to keep it simple. My plan encompasses the best from many plans. You can adapt it to fit any ethnic or cultural cuisine and you can use this eating plan the rest of your life. No foods are restricted, but some need to be significantly reduced. I would suggest that if you like this plan, start your weight loss journey by printing the following diagram and place it on your refrigerator.

Living for A Healthy Heart Plan

- **Eat**
  - o a plant-based diet of more fruits and vegetables.
  - o whole grains, beans and dark rice.
  - o lean meats the size of a deck of cards no more than twice a day.
  - o lower fat dairy products such as skim milk.
  - o olive or canola oil.
  - o palm size of nuts a day for one snack.

- **Reduce**
  - o processed foods and saturated fats in your diet.
  - o desserts and sugary drinks.
  - o salt.
  - o alcohol.
  - o portion sizes.

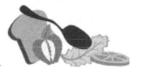

- **Hydrate**
  - o by drinking more water.

Remember to be realistic, start small, and go slow. Don't try and eat all of these healthy things at once. It may be too much. Be realistic about what you can change. Follow Wansink's approach in *Mindless Eating* and *Slim By Design* and set your environment up for success (SlimByDesign.org). Food is important to your quality of life. All changes help. Your job is to decide just how much you are able to do. The choice remains with you.

Healthier Eating for the Family

Some people are highly motivated to make changes in their eating but run into a brick wall with their spouse or children. It took your family a long time to get out of balance and it will take a long time to get it back. Be the role model that they need you to be. As they see the changes in you, they will be more likely to come around. Be sure that your home environment is set up to be successful. Prepare healthier meals and limit the availability of the junk food that is left around the house.

Personal Story

I had a friend whose husband was a police officer. He was called to a home where he witnessed a young child choke and die from a piece of hotdog. He instructed his wife to keep their child on baby food until she was at least three years old. The little girl grew up without getting used to the taste of crunchy vegetables or fresh fruit. She craved soft and squishy foods. As a teenager, she was profoundly obese with a BMI of 44. What started out as well meaning had untoward traumatic consequences.

On the other hand, another relative of mine was a busy athlete. In high school, he had a 1,500 calorie a day deficit during basketball season. He was burning his calories and too thin. It was hard to give him the nutrition that he needed as he was running for hours each day. Daily protein milkshakes were given to increase his caloric intake. What a problem to have! He also loved junk food. I noticed that if the family ran out of cookies or chips, he reached for the yogurt and fruit. He continued consuming high calories into adulthood. When the activity levels and physical growth decreased, the weight increased dramatically. As an adult, he struggles with maintaining a healthy weight. His excess weight is coming off, but it isn't easy. Teach your children good nutrition. If the junk isn't around, they may squawk, but they will eventually reach for the healthier food. Good nutrition is better for everyone!

Sweeteners

High Fructose Corn Syrup

Recently, there has been a growing debate on whether high fructose corn syrup (HFCS) is harmful and a leading cause of obesity. Critics argue that since high fructose corn syrup (HFCS) began to replace cane sugar in many processed foods in the 1980s, it must be the cause of the rising obesity epidemic.[27]

The fructose in HFCS is twice as sweet as cane sugar and is broken down in the liver whereas cane sugar readily enters the blood. Cane sugar stimulates the release of insulin, which triggers the release of leptin an appetite suppressant. Critics argue that HFCS may stimulate ghrelin, a chemical which increases hunger.

Experts from the Academy of Nutrition and Dietetics examined the current body of research and published the following statement:[28]

> These studies consistently found little evidence that HFCS differs uniquely from sucrose (cane sugar) and other nutritive sweeteners in metabolic effects (i.e., circulating glucose, insulin, postprandial (after eating) triglycerides, leptin and ghrelin), subjective effects (i.e., hunger, satiety, and energy intake at subsequent meals) and adverse effect such as risk of weight gain. Randomized trials dealing specifically with HFCS were of limited numbers, short duration, and of small sample size; therefore, long-term data are needed. (749)

According to their report, a sugar is a sugar once it gets into your blood, but more research is needed. It may be that there is a connection between the greater use of HFCS and obesity, but during the rise in consumption of HFCS, portion sizes also increased dramatically. I think that the increase in portion size probably plays a larger role in the obesity epidemic, but who really knows. Caution is called for in this situation. Limit all of your HFCS and cane sugar intake for a variety of health reasons. The American Heart Association recommends that women reduce their sugar content to less than 100 calories a day and men less than 150 calories a day.[29] While these guidelines are helpful, most Americans will find them too challenging to follow. Less is best so reduce your overall sugar consumption whenever you can.

Artificial Sweeteners

Another controversy that has arisen is the use of artificial sweeteners. There are many types of artificial sweeteners, which do "not" raise blood sugar levels. They taste many times sweeter than cane sugar, natural sugars found in fruits, and HFCS. Susan Swithers from the Department of Psychological Sciences and Ingestive Behavior Research from Purdue University hypothesizes that the brain learns to react differently when presented with artificial sweeteners that do not result in an expected increase in blood sugar.[30]

> In lots of ways (artificial sweeteners) have been given the benefit of the doubt just because they don't have any calories…What happens when you have a sweetener is you get the sweet taste but calories and sugar don't show up. Your body says, "Wait this isn't what I was expecting to happen," and over time you may not produce those same anticipatory responses. Blunting those responses could cause people to overeat and experience consistently higher blood sugar levels, which could potentially lead to the onset of type 2 diabetes.

The experts from the Academy of Nutrition and Dietetics organization reviewed artificial sweeteners and stated:[28]

> Consumers who want a sweet taste… can choose from seven FDA-approved NNS [non-nutritive sweeteners

(artificial sweeteners)] based on their personal taste preference and the intended use (e.g., for cooking or for tabletop use) NNS, when substituted for nutritive sweeteners (HFCS or cane sugar), may help... manage blood glucose or weight. (754)

FDA-Approved Artificial Sweeteners[31]

Sweetener	Common Name
Acesulfame Potassium (K)	Sunett, Sweet One
Aspartame	Nutrasweet, Equal
Neotame	Not available
Saccharin	Sweet' N Low, Sweet Twin, Sugar Twin
Sucralose	Splenda
Stevia/Rebaudioside	A Sweet Leaf
*American Diabetes Association	

Artificial sweeteners are required for persons with diabetes who desire the joy of sweet food without dangerously increasing their blood sugar. I would refer all of you with diabetes to speak with your healthcare provider or diabetes dietitian regarding the use of sweeteners and medications. However, everyone else should use caution regarding artificial sweeteners. Far too many people who struggle with weight consume several diet drinks per day. They think that since the drinks have zero calories, they can consume unlimited amounts. In truth, no one knows the full impact of artificial sweeteners over long-term health. I would encourage you to consider limiting your consumption of these products to less than one a day and switch to unsweetened sparkling seltzer water. More research is needed.

Alcohol

Alcohol consumption can also contribute to weight gain. It is often used to lift a negative mood and calories accumulate very quickly. A 4-ounce glass of red wine contains 85 calories, while sweet dessert wine has 181 calories.[32] A 12-ounce serving of light beer contains 100 calories, while dark beer may contain up to 160 calories. A 1.5 ounce of vodka, rum, or whiskey (80 to 100 proof) has a caloric content that ranges between 95 to 124 calories. People often ingest more junk foods and calories when drinking alcohol. If you have too much and a hangover ensues, you may reach for higher fatty junk foods to relieve the symptoms. It's a vicious cycle and must be controlled for weight loss. Alcohol is converted to triglycerides and, if not burned for fuel, will be stored as body fat. Wansink shared a wonderful story about a man who lost weight by changing from beer to red wine. When asked why it worked, the man stated that he didn't like red wine so he consumed less.[8]

Orlistat (Anti-Obesity Drug)

If your BMI is greater than 30 or greater than 27 with medical problems related to your obesity, the drug Orlistat may be helpful.[5] It works by reducing fat absorption by 30 percent.[33] This medication only results in less than 5 to 10 percent weight loss with very annoying side effects in most people.[33] Unfortunately, the weight will return when the medication is discontinued. It requires taking the medication within ninety minutes of a meal three times a day.[34] If you consume a diet high in fats, the side effects will be more pronounced which include gas, oily stools, and abdominal pain. It must be used with caution in people with gallbladder disease.

Medical research continues to look for more effective weight loss medications. Drugs to increase leptin, which would decrease appetite, are an exciting area of research. Some antidepressants have been found to decrease appetite as well. I will refer you to your healthcare provider for questions related to obesity medications. If a pharmaceutical company could find a medication to help people lose weight, they would make billions, but to date, they haven't been successful. Nothing replaces a healthier diet and more activity.

Bariatric Surgery

If your BMI is greater than 40 or greater than 35 with obesity related medical problems, you may be a candidate for bariatric surgery.[5] Bariatric surgery works by decreasing your stomach size. Less food may enter the stomach, you feel fuller and lose weight. There are several different types of procedures. When considering this surgery, you have to ask yourself, "What are the benefits versus the risks of the surgery? Have I exhausted a variety of weight loss strategies such as taking antidepressants, restricting calories, increasing physical activity, and they have not worked? Is my severe obesity causing me serious weight-related complications?" If yes, you may wish to speak with your healthcare provider about the procedure. In my experience, physicians have become more supportive of the surgery especially for their patients who are suffering from deadly weight-related complications.

Take Away Points

From prehistoric times, the taste of sugar has helped us to distinguish sweet edible berries from sour poisonous ones. Salt allowed us to retain water, preventing dehydration and fat sustained us on long hunter-gatherer journeys.[8] Our biology craves the very foods that can increase our weight. Is it any wonder that sedentary modern men and women struggle with excess weight? However, maintaining a healthy weight can be done.

Jennie's Top 10 List for Successful Weight Loss

#10	Increase your physical activity.
#9	Weigh yourself frequently and adjust eating as needed.
#8	Eat a 100 calorie snack for dessert to satisfy a craving.
#7	Order a kids meal or share an entrée.
#6	Watch your portion sizes.
#5	Use a smaller plate.
#4	Eat more fruits and vegetables.
#3	Don't skip meals.
#2	Treat a negative mood state.
And the #1 Top Tip for Successful Weight Loss Is: KEEP BUSY-AVOID BOREDOM!	

I hope that this chapter provided you with a new way of thinking about weight loss and simple strategies for success. If you have special dietary needs or you are down to less than thirty pounds to lose, a dietitian may take you the rest of the way. There is no doubt that obesity will soon overcome smoking as the more dangerous risk factor for a heart attack and stroke.[1] It is imperative that you begin to consider how to change your life now. Keep it simple, stick with it, and set up your environment for success. The simple strategies from this chapter will help you get there. Changing is hard, but you can do it!

Additional Information:

American Heart Association (Dining Out)   http://www.heart.org/HEARTORG/GettingHealthy/NutritionCenter/DiningOut/Dining-Out-Tips-by-Cuisine_UCM_308333_Article.jsp.

National Heart Lung and Blood Institute (NHLBI) (Portion Distortion Quiz) http://www.nhlbi.nih.gov/health/educatio nal/wecan/eat-right/portion-distortion.htm.

Nutrition.gov http://www.nutrition.gov/.

Obesity Initiative NHLBI) http://www.nhlbi.nih.gov/health/ public/heart/index.htm#obesity.

To cease smoking is the easiest thing I ever did;
I ought to know because I've done it a thousand times.

—American Author, Mark Twain

7

Strategies to Help End a Tobacco Habit

If you are a smoker or use a smokeless tobacco product, you are not a bad person. Somewhere along the way, you tried a tobacco product, and it didn't take long to become addicted to nicotine. You try and quit, but the cravings sabotage your best efforts. Well-meaning healthcare providers, families, and friends often worsen the problem with an ineffective approach that makes you feel defensive and stigmatized. My approach is summed up in the following phrase, "I'm not here to beat you up about your smoking but rather provide you with information that other smokers found helpful when they quit."

This chapter will get you started thinking about your options. However, I highly recommend that you follow up with an expert smoking cessation counselor to walk you through the quitting process. The phone call will help you whether you are just beginning to think about quitting or very committed to quitting. Their phone numbers and information are provided at the end of this chapter. Finally, smoking is a pleasurable activity. Why would anyone quit "if they didn't have to." Even though everyone knows that smoking is bad, parts of this chapter will provide you with a new way of thinking about your habit in order to enhance your motivation to quit. This chapter will help loved ones and healthcare providers better understand the physiology of tobacco addiction and strategies that are the most effective in cessation. I begin with some background information on tobacco use.

Overview of the Problem

Smoking is one of the most challenging addictions to conquer. The damage from smoking not only shortens the life of the smoker but also the nonsmoker exposed to the secondhand smoke. Approximately 480,000 Americans die each year from smoking related diseases.[1] It is the equivalent of half of the passengers on a cruise ship such as the Queen Mary 2 dying each day.[2] We have become immune to these numbers. Due to the severe obstacle of nicotine addiction, denial remains a major problem. However, 70 percent of smokers want to quit smoking, half tried to quit, and two thirds of those who relapsed want to try and quit again.[3] Today, half of all people who ever smoked have quit.[3] The motivation appears to be high. The question remains, "Why is it so hard to quit?"

In my experience, tobacco users underestimate the power of their addiction to nicotine, which actually changes the way that the brain functions. If you use a tobacco product and want to be successful at quitting, you will need to think differently about your problem and be open to a variety of quitting strategies. Nicotine addiction is a very complex problem and requires multiple strategies. I've found that most tobacco users are unaware of all the resources available to help them become a successful quitter. It's also important to know that many people have been snared into a nicotine addiction. The manufacturers of the products utilize a great deal of cunning to get you hooked and coming back to buy more. I think it will help you to understand the history of how tobacco use expanded on American shores.

Tobacco Use in America[4]

Tobacco is a native indigenous plant commonly found on the North American continent. The Mayans were the first to use the *Nicotania tabacum* plant for chewing and smoking. Rodriguez de Jerez, a member of the 1492 Christopher Columbus expedition, observed Indians enjoying the smoking of dried tobacco leaves wrapped with palm leaves or corn husks. Upon returning to Europe, he was arrested for smoking the product. They thought he was possessed by evil and imprisoned him for seven years. By the time he was released, smoking had spread throughout Spain and into Europe. In 1561, a Frenchman Jean Nicot de Villemain described the "mind altering" substance contained within tobacco that he labeled nicotine. In the 1600s, American colonists realized the value of exported tobacco growing in their fields. It was said that Napoleon was so addicted to snuff that he used seven pounds a month. Snuff is ground tobacco leaves snorted into the nose or a pinch placed inside the gums of the mouth.

The first cigarette was created by an Egyptian soldier in the 1830s who stuffed tobacco into a paper tube made to hold gunpowder. After the Civil War, returning Union soldiers brought their new smoking habit back to the north. By the end of the nineteenth century, cigarettes and cigars were the more popular form of tobacco use. Cigarettes were placed in the food rations of soldiers fighting in both World War I and II. General John Pershing stated, "Tobacco is as indispensible as the daily ration; we must have thousands of tons without delay" (p. 1037).[4] Soldiers brought the habit back to their homeland where it exploded. By 1949, half of men and one-third of women were smokers. The following chart displays how tobacco consumption changed over time.

Adult Smoking Rates Over Time

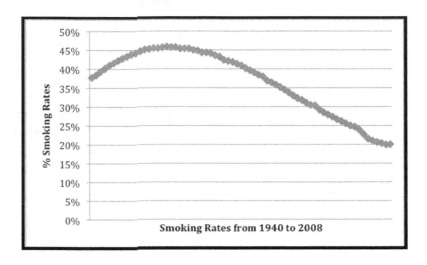

*Center for Disease Control and Prevention Data

As the smoking research accumulated, the landmark 1964 "Surgeon General Report on Smoking and Health" was released by surgeon general Dr. Luther Terry.[1] The public was notified of the dangerous link between smoking and cancer risk. The report had a dramatic impact on smokers and began to change smoking rates. In the 1970's, cigarette advertisements were prohibited on public television and smoking was banned from buses and airlines. The cost has increased dramatically primarily due to tax hikes. Today, a pack of cigarettes range from $4.96 in Kentucky to $14.50 in New York.[5] Many factors have influenced the decline in smoking rates. Escalating costs, the stigma of smoking, bans in public places, awareness of the harm from smoking, and treatments to augment cessation have played a major role.

Americans are getting much closer to the Healthy People 2020 goal of a smoking rate less than 12 percent.[1] Today 18 percent of adults over the age of 18 are smokers.[1]

Tobacco Products

Various tobacco products are available that contain the addictive ingredient nicotine: cigarettes, bidis, e-cigarettes, cigars, and smokeless tobacco.

Cigarettes

The cigarette is a highly engineered device that rapidly delivers the drug nicotine to the brain, killing half of all long term users.[1] When burned, 7,000 chemicals are created of which many are known to cause cancer.[1]

Chemicals Found in a Cigarette

Acetone	Found in nail polish remover.
Acetic Acid	Ingredient in hair dye.
Ammonia	Household cleaner.
Arsenic	Used in rat poison.
Benzene	Found in rubber cement.
Butane	Used in lighter fluid.
Cadmium	Active component of battery acid.
Carbon Monoxide	Released in car exhaust fumes.
Formaldehyde	Embalming fluid.
Hexamine	Found in barbecue lighter fluid.
Lead	Used in batteries.
Naphthalene	An ingredient in moth balls.
Methanol	A main component in rocket fuel.
Nicotine	Used as insecticide.
Tar	Material for paving roads.
Toluene	Used to manufacture paint.
*American Lung Association	

Within ten to fifteen seconds from a puff on a cigarette, nicotine floods the "feel-good" center of the brain and releases dopamine, which causes very pleasant sensations.[6] This rapid positive benefit occurs because the smoke is drawn into the lungs where it comes in contact with the rich blood supply and is immediately pumped to the brain. Adrenalin is simultaneously released which increases the heart rate, blood pressure, and blood sugar. The smoker feels both more relaxed and more awake. The immediate dopamine and adrenalin release is the main problem with breaking the cycle of the nicotine addiction.

A typical smoker takes ten puffs off a single cigarette.[6] The amount of nicotine absorbed varies depending on how deeply the smoke is drawn into the lungs and the amount of nicotine contained within the cigarette. Peak concentration of nicotine in the blood occurs after seven to eight minutes. Smokers puff to maintain the higher nicotine levels and the drug effect. A pack a day smoker gets about 200 hits of nicotine each day.[6] Interestingly, smokers who switch to a lower nicotine product often maintain the same nicotine levels by inhaling more deeply on the new product. With any chronic use of a tobacco product, the brain changes to adapt to increasing amounts of nicotine.

The Myth of Social Smoking

Many social or light smokers do not label themselves as a "smoker" because they do not smoke on a daily basis, smoke only one to three cigarettes a day or a few a week. This troubling perception occurs with social or light cigar and smokeless tobacco users as well. When asked if they smoke or use tobacco, they often deny it to family, friends, and their healthcare provider. Cigar smokers rationalize their use, "I do not inhale." Light tobacco users do not view their habit as harmful, "I can take it or leave it. I'm not addicted."

Unfortunately, any amount of smoking or tobacco use increases the stickiness of the blood, damages the arterial lining, and increases risk for a heart attack, stroke, cancer, or several other diseases. According to the American Heart Association Statistical Update 2013, "There is no evidence to date that reducing the amount smoked by smoking fewer cigarettes per day reduces the risk for cardiovascular disease" (e61).[7] Don't be fooled by this social smoking mythology. If you use a tobacco product, no matter the amount, you are increasing your risk for untoward harmful health outcomes.

Bidi Cigarettes

Bidis are flavored cigarettes that come from India and have become popular with teenagers. They can be purchased individually and come in a variety of candy flavors: chocolate, cherry, strawberry, licorice, and orange. Because they are advertised as more "natural" than cigarettes, some think that they are safer. However, bidis deliver three to five times more nicotine than regular cigarettes and are unfiltered.[8] They are a gateway tobacco product for other forms of tobacco use.

A Word about E-Cigarettes

E-cigarettes have been available for the past ten years. A battery-operated device warms a vapor that delivers nicotine during the inhalation of the product. It has not been available long enough to study whether this nicotine device is a helpful invention or a health problem. Proponents say it offers the nicotine fix and the sensation of smoking without the tar and is a helpful aide when quitting smoking. Opponents are concerned that it glamorizes smoking and may be a gateway to traditional smoking. Some are candy flavored, which seems to be enticing to the youth. The vapors are an irritant and it is unknown whether this will damage the lung of the user or whether there are more secondhand repercussions.

The Centers for Disease Control (CDC), the World Health Organization (WHO), and the American Heart Association (AHA) have issued concerns regarding the growing use of e-cigarettes among teens. Dr. Tim McAfee, director of the CDC Office on Smoking and Health stated:[9]

> We are very concerned about nicotine use among our youth, regardless of whether it comes from conventional cigarettes, e-cigarettes or other tobacco products. Not only is nicotine highly addictive, it can harm adolescent brain development.

The WHO have called for a ban on e-cigarette use indoors and restrictions to minors as the fruit, candy, and alcohol-flavored products are especially enticing to teens.[10] Nancy Brown, CEO of the American Heart Association, stated:[11]

> Recent studies raise concerns that e-cigarettes may be a gateway to traditional tobacco products for the nation's youth, and could renormalize smoking in our society. These disturbing developments have helped convince the association that e-cigarettes need to be strongly regulated, thoroughly researched and closely monitored.

You may refer to the American Heart Association policy statement on e-cigarettes by visiting www.americanheart.org.

From my perspective, it is known that nicotine is highly addictive and its toxicity may become a problem. I don't see how this product would be helpful for smoking cessation if used for over six months and e-cigarettes are becoming a gateway smoking addiction for youth. You may be substituting one addictive behavior for another. Most importantly, it does not change the hand-to-mouth habit associated with smoking. I do not recommend this product for those reasons.

Cigars

Many people think that cigars are somewhat safer to smoke than cigarettes, but this is also a myth. A cigar is tobacco wrapped with a tobacco leaf while a cigarette is tobacco wrapped with paper. One large cigar contains as much tobacco as an entire pack of cigarettes. While a cigarette contains 8 mg of nicotine delivering between 1 mg to 2 mg, a cigar contains between 100 mg and 200 mg with some approaching 444 mg of nicotine.[12] The amount that gets into the system depends on the size and type of cigar smoked, whether the cigar is inhaled, how many puffs are taken, and how long it is smoked which can take between one to two hours. Cigar smokers keep the burning cigar in their mouth, allowing the nicotine to be absorbed through the mucous membranes of the mouth. The cigar smoke dissolves quickly when it comes in contact with saliva. If the cigar is inhaled, it will reach the brain as quickly as with cigarette smoking due to the fast absorption in the lungs. The secondhand smoke particulates from a cigar linger in the air for hours longer than cigarette smoke. The cigar carries greater risk for oral cancers as the cigar is held in the mouth longer.

Smokeless Tobacco

Approximately 3.5 percent of people over twelve years of age use a smokeless tobacco product. About 46 percent of new users begin their habit in high school, where 11 percent of males and 1.5 percent of females use smokeless tobacco.[13] Moist snuff is finely ground tobacco that is placed between the lower lip or cheek and gum. Chewing tobacco is also placed between the cheek, gum or teeth and can be chewed. Sugar is added to the products to enhance the taste. The user spits out the soaked tobacco. With either smokeless product, nicotine is absorbed through the mucous membranes of the mouth. Dry snuff is a powder that is sniffed or inhaled into the nose.

The absorption of nicotine is much slower with smokeless tobacco compared to rapid inhalation into the lungs from smoking. Patients have told me that it can take up to twenty minutes, but eventually produces similar effects of relaxation and greater wakefulness. It is an easier addiction to hide since no smoke is produced.

Danger of Tobacco Use

Inhaled Tobacco

In chapter 1, I described the development of plaque and how it leads to a heart attack and stroke. Inhaled tobacco causes serious damage to the inside lining of all of your arteries throughout the body. As you inhale the product, it is quickly carried deep into the lungs. Normally, oxygen binds to the hemoglobin on the waiting blood cell and transported to the tissues of the body. When burning a tobacco product, carbon monoxide is produced, which is similar to the exhaust from a car. The carbon monoxide takes the place of oxygen. Anywhere from 3 percent to 15 percent of the oxygen on the hemoglobin will be replaced with carbon monoxide.[14] That amount may not sound like much, but it is toxic to the arteries as it travels through the blood. The toxins within the smoke are pumped into the heart and out to the rest of the body. The areas that receive the greatest exposure from the toxins are damaged the most, but the problem occurs throughout the body.

The damage to the arteries causes plaque build-up and leads to a heart attack and stroke. Each time you take a puff on a cigarette or cigar, chew or snuff smokeless tobacco, your blood pressure, heart rate, and blood sugar increase. High blood pressure causes a sandpaper effect on the inside lining damaging the artery. The excess sugar scratches the lining, making the problem worse. Instead of the artery being nice and smooth like the inside of your cheek, it is rough and irritated. LDL (bad) cholesterol traveling in the blood gets caught in the rougher areas and plaque begins to build up.

Another complication from smoking is that the blood becomes very sticky. It can clump together. Recall that in a heart attack, you take an aspirin to reduce the clumping and size of the blood clot that is forming and blocking the artery. If your blood is already sticky, this clumping will occur faster and the clot will become larger and the problem will be much worse. An interesting study that examined 902 heart attack patients found that the blood clot formed during a heart attack was larger the closer the event occurred to the last cigarette smoked.[15] Damaged arteries can also cause the loss of limbs due to amputees, facial premature aging or wrinkles, hearing loss, and impotence.

The entire body is vulnerable and easily damaged from the exposure to the toxins, which explains why cancer development is so widespread. Whatever the toxins touch becomes irritated and damaged. Think of where the contaminated air flows: mouth and nose, through the throat, down the windpipe, into the bronchial airways, into the lungs, pumped through the heart, and then transported throughout all of the organs of the body. Your risk for developing cancer depends upon your genetic vulnerability to cancer and your exposure to other toxins within the environment.

Secondhand Smoke

Throughout this book, I have made the point that lifestyle choices, including continued tobacco use, are your choices to make. However, you must also be aware of how your behavior impacts others who choose not to smoke. I think this information will help increase your motivation to quit smoking, especially learning how it impacts children.

For a long time, the danger from secondhand smoke went unrecognized. It is estimated that 49,000 nonsmokers die from exposure to secondhand smoke each year[7] and of those, 3,000 died from lung cancer.[16] Adults exposed to secondhand smoke for even brief periods have stickier blood, damage to their arterial linings as previously described, decreased blood flow, increased risk for a heart attack, stroke, and various cancers.[16] Children exposed to secondhand smoke have additional risks such as sudden infant death syndrome (SIDS), respiratory and ear infections, and asthma.

Secondhand smoke is a mixture of gases and small particles that are dispersed into the air when burning a tobacco product. It contains hundreds of chemicals which are toxic and many known to cause cancer.[16] Nonsmokers inhale the unfiltered smoke most commonly at home or previously in the workplace. Restaurants, bars, apartments, and cars are other places of exposure. Some mistakenly believe that if you have a strong enough air cleaner system you can remove the harmful toxins from the contaminated air. The Surgeon General Report of 2006 contained the following statement regarding the potential to remove the secondhand smoke from the environment:[16]

> Conventional air cleaning systems can remove large particles, but not the smaller particles or the gases found in secondhand smoke. Routine operation of a heating, ventilating, and air conditioning system can distribute secondhand smoke throughout a building. The American Society of Heating, Refrigerating and Air-Conditioning Engineers (ASHRAE), the preeminent U.S. body on ventilation issues, has concluded that ventilation technology cannot be relied on to control health risks from secondhand smoke exposure. (4)

Cotinine is a byproduct formed from the breakdown of nicotine in the body and is detected in saliva, blood, or urine.[16] Cotinine levels in the blood have been decreasing as smoke-free environments have increased and smoking rates have declined. Between 1999 and 2000, 52 percent of adult nonsmokers had cotinine detected in the blood, while between 2007 and 2008, the number had decreased to 40 percent.[7] During that same time frame, children had similar reductions in cotinine levels. Interestingly, data from the CDC estimated that between 2007 and 2008, 18 percent of children lived in homes where someone smoked[17], but 54 percent had detectable cotinine levels[1] If only 18 percent of children live in smoking homes, one has to wonder where the other children are being exposed to secondhand smoke.

Researchers found that if children lived with nonsmokers but in an apartment building where other tenants smoked, 45 percent had detectable cotinine levels.[17] It was getting to them through the ventilation system. Restaurants where smoking was allowed were other locations of exposure. Presumably, the children were seated in nonsmoking areas but were still getting the toxins in their system. This information led to some of the public bans implemented across the nation.

Thirdhand Smoke

I wanted to make you aware of research that is ongoing related to thirdhand smoke. According to the 2006 Surgeon General's Report:[16]

> Thirdhand smoke is particles and gases given off by cigarettes that cling to walls, clothes and even hair and skin. Some early studies have shown that babies of parents who smoke only outside had cotinine levels seven times higher than in the infants of non-smokers. (5)

Smokeless Tobacco

Another common misconception is that snuff or chewing tobacco is safer than cigarettes or cigars since they are not burned. The danger from smokeless tobacco is that it remains in one place for a long time, irritating the tissues and thus increasing risk for cancer. The abrasives within the products lead to microscopic irritation and bleeding of the gums, which allows for greater absorption of nicotine.

Complications from Smokeless Tobacco

Mouth, tongue, cheek, gum and throat cancer.
Cancer of the esophagus.
Stomach cancer.
Pancreatic cancer.
Heart attack and strokes.
Addiction to nicotine-progressing to smoking.
Leukoplakia-precancerous white sores in the mouth.
Receding gums.
Bone loss around the roots of the teeth.
Abrasion of the teeth and gums.
Cavities and tooth decay.
Tooth loss.
Stained and colored teeth.
Bad breath.
*American Cancer Society

The smokeless tobacco available in the United States has very high levels of cancer-causing substances called carcinogens. It is estimated that three out of four daily users have early precancerous mouth lesions from contact with the toxins within the product.[13]

Hopefully, this information has enhanced your motivation to stop smoking. "Why would a reasonable person give up a habit that they love if they didn't have to?" In the next section, I describe the payoffs of smoking. These powerful influences on smoking behavior are the main reason why it is so difficult to quit. As you consider quitting, you will need to rethink how you will cope with these barriers. I will follow with the benefits of quitting, which not surprisingly is a much longer list.

Payoffs of Tobacco Use

Avoid Withdrawal Symptoms

Probably the main reason why tobacco use of any kind is so addictive is the annoying withdrawal symptoms that occur when nicotine levels decrease. The symptoms subside as soon as a tobacco product is used. Within a few seconds for smokers and several minutes for cigar, snuff, or chewing tobacco users, nicotine breaks through the blood brain barrier and stimulates the release of dopamine. Withdrawal symptoms are immediately eliminated.

Stimulant

Nicotine also works as a stimulant increasing heart rate and blood pressure. If you are feeling sluggish and you have a cigarette, cigar, or smokeless tobacco product, you feel more awake, alert and energized.

Less Peer Pressure/Self-Esteem

If surrounded by others who smoke, life is much less complicated if you maintain your tobacco habit. My parents began heavy smoking habits in order to fit in with the adults around them. Teenagers are especially vulnerable to peer pressure, but athletes and adults are impacted too. Media plays a role as teens are more likely to smoke if they see movie heroes or heroines smoke.[1] Smoking may make you feel more like you fit in and builds your self-esteem. These payoffs while few are some of the main obstacles in quitting.

Benefits of Quitting Tobacco Use

As you can see, there are a multitude of benefits for quitting tobacco use. Some of them will occur immediately upon quitting. In order to become a successful quitter, you will need to learn healthier substitutes for nicotine and employ a variety of cessation strategies.

Benefits from Quitting

Overall improved health throughout the entire body.
Food will taste better.
Improved sense of smell.
Save money.
Feeling better about yourself.
Home, car, clothing and breath will smell better.
Set a good example for your children.
Have healthier babies and children.
Feel better physically.
Improved appearance with less wrinkling.
Whiter teeth.
*Treating Tobacco Use and Dependence *U.S. Department of Health and Human Services*

Each person will respond to smoking cessation differently.

Timeline of Smoking Cessation

After 20 Minutes	Heart rate and blood pressure decreases.
2 Hours	Blood pressure returns to pre-tobacco use levels. Temperature in the hands and feet return to normal. Withdrawal symptoms begin: cravings, anxiety, drowsiness or trouble sleeping, increased appetite.
After 12 Hours	Carbon monoxide levels in the blood drop to normal levels while oxygen levels increase.
After 24 Hours	Your chance of an immediate heart attack begins to decrease.
After 48 Hours	Smell and taste begin to return as nerves heal.
After 3 Days	Nicotine is out of the body and withdrawal symptoms have peaked. Symptoms such as headache, nausea, cramps, and anxiety may worsen. Reward yourself for getting this far!
2 to 3 Weeks	Shortness of breath is decreasing, circulation improving.
Within 3 Months	Your circulation improves and lung function increases up to 30%.
1 to 9 Months	Lungs begin to repair. The tiny cilia hairs in lungs return to normal. Most withdrawal symptoms are gone.
After 1 Year	The risk of a heart attack is half that of a current smoker.
After 5 Years	Your stroke risk is reduced to that of a nonsmoker.
After 10 Years	The lung cancer death rate is about half that of a current smoker. The risk of cancer of the mouth, throat, esophagus, bladder, kidney and pancreas decreases.
After 15 Years	The risk of heart disease is the same as a nonsmoker.
*American Cancer Society	

Overcoming Your Nicotine Addiction

Many tobacco users remain in denial regarding whether or not they believe that they have an addiction to nicotine. The American Psychological Association (APA) defines addiction as:[18]

> Addiction is a condition in which the body must have a drug to avoid physical and psychological withdrawal symptoms. Addiction's first stage is dependence, during which the search for a drug dominates an individual's life. An addict eventually develops tolerance, which forces the person to consume larger and larger doses of the drug to get the same effect.

I think that most would agree that nicotine fits the APA definition. Further, the Surgeon General Report from 1988 stated that nicotine was as addictive as heroine and cocaine.[19] People who are addicted to nicotine use tobacco to elevate their mood, become more alert, enhance concentration, or avoid withdrawal symptoms.

The withdrawal symptoms begin within a few hours of cessation and reach a peak within one to two weeks.[20] However, in my experience, people complain of cravings off and on for months, but the symptoms do diminish over time. Some of the more common withdrawal symptoms are irritability, anxiety, insomnia, difficulty concentrating, restlessness, and depressive thoughts related to decreasing blood levels of nicotine.[6] The central nervous system is depressed. Heart rate and blood pressure decrease leading to prolonged drowsiness, depressive symptoms, constipation, and headache. Blood sugar levels are lower so appetite is increased.

Nicotine Blood Levels

During sleep, nicotine blood levels plummet. Upon awakening, the smoker begins to smoke to raise nicotine levels. If unencumbered, smoking occurs more frequently in the morning until nicotine blood levels are elevated. Throughout the rest of the day, smoking slows down but keeps a pace to maintain the higher nicotine blood levels. The cycle repeats the next day.

Nicotine Addiction Quiz

Yes	No	Do you smoke your first cigarette within 30 minutes of waking up in the morning?
Yes	No	Do you smoke 20 cigarettes (one pack) or more each day?
Yes	No	At times when you can't smoke or don't have any cigarettes, do you feel a craving for one?
Yes	No	Is it tough to keep from smoking for more than a few hours?
Yes	No	When you are sick enough to stay in bed, do you still smoke?
If you answer yes to 2 of these questions you are addicted to nicotine.		
*American Lung Association, 7 Steps To A Smoke-free Life, 1998		

Conquering the nicotine addiction is the *most* important step in successfully quitting. Everything must be utilized to help you quit! Smoking cessation medications along with behavior change strategies double the quit rates.[20] The following is a discussion of the medications that help curb the addiction to nicotine and help you become more successful at quitting. These are rough guidelines. You should work with your smoking counselor, pharmacist and healthcare provider for the best dose and medication appropriate for you.

Nicotine Replacements

Nicotine replacement medications are not designed to completely stop the withdrawal symptoms of tobacco cessation. They do not reach as high a nicotine blood level as smoking but reduce the cravings and take the edge off of the cravings. Some products are generally not recommended for patients who are recovering from a heart attack or pregnant women. Speak with your healthcare provider about whether you are a candidate for any of the following medications and how you should take them.

Patch[6]

The patch is an over-the-counter nicotine replacement product that is placed on the skin and provides a slow release of nicotine. It takes two to six hours to begin to feel relief and once removed the effects diminish. Speak with your smoking counselor, pharmacist, or healthcare provider regarding the appropriate patch for you. The benefit of the patch is that the oral hand to mouth habit is not reinforced as with other nicotine replacement medications. The twenty-four-hour patch avoids morning drops in nicotine levels which may trigger cravings and relapse. Side effects from the patch may include insomnia and skin irritation. The patch site should be rotated and each site should not be used again for one week. Trouble sleeping may indicate a dose that is too high while withdrawal symptoms may indicate a dose that is too low. According to the *Quick Reference Guide for Clinicians 2008 Update: Treating Tobacco Use and Dependence,* the patch is safe to use for cardiac patients.[20] However, if you have a history of cardiac problems, you should check with your healthcare provider before using this medication.

Gum[6]

Using over-the-counter nicotine gum "improves smoking cessation rates between 40 percent to 60 percent compared with controls through 12 months of follow-up."[6] (178) The nicotine medication is released during chewing. The gum is chewed five to eight times until a peppery taste appears, then parked inside the cheek. When a craving returns, the process is repeated. Chewing too quickly may produce nausea, throat irritation, and hiccups. Peak levels of nicotine are reached within thirty minutes. Acidic foods such as coffee, soft drinks, or juice should be avoided fifteen minutes before, during, and after nicotine gum use. The dose varies depending upon your tobacco use, and the mint flavor is preferred by most people. Speak with your smoking counselor, pharmacist, or healthcare provider regarding the appropriate dose for you.

Lozenge[6]

The lozenge comes in 2 mg and 4 mg doses. If you seek a cigarette within the first thirty minutes upon waking, you are more addicted to nicotine and need the larger dose for withdrawal relief. Again, speak with your smoking counselor, pharmacist, or healthcare provider regarding the appropriate dose for you. The lozenge dissolves in the mouth within twenty to thirty minutes when peak nicotine levels are reached. The lozenge will not work effectively if chewed. You should not eat or drink for fifteen minutes before or while the lozenge is dissolving. You may feel a tingling sensation in your mouth. Dosages should be tapered before discontinuing the medication.

Inhaler[6]

The inhaler is a prescription used to inhale nicotine into the lungs for roughly twenty minutes and is equivalent to the amount of nicotine in two cigarettes. Side effects may include coughing, mouth and throat irritation, and indigestion. One problem with using the inhaler is that it doesn't break the hand to mouth habit associated with smoking.

Nasal Spray[6]

The prescription nasal spray delivers rapid nicotine relief. The spray should not be inhaled, swallowed, or sniffed. The dose is generally one to two sprays in each nostril per hour not exceeding five sprays per hour. Peak nicotine levels are reached within four to fifteen minutes. It is the most effective nicotine replacement product recommended for heavy smokers. Side effects may include irritation of the nose and throat, increased blood pressure, and heart rhythm irregularities. Use of the spray may cause a head rush of dopamine or good feelings similar to smoking, which can be addicting. The product should not be used any longer than three months.

Other Smoking Cessation Medications

Bupropion (Zyban)[6]

Zyban is the only antidepressant approved by the FDA for smoking cessation. Depressive and anxious moods are a common problem during tobacco cessation along with fears of weight gain. The average weight gain during smoking cessation is five pounds. While testing Zyban as an antidepressant, it was discovered that it also reduced cravings for smoking and appetite. The medication helps smokers quit and they do not gain as much weight.

The medication must be started one to two weeks before the quit date. You begin by taking 150 mg daily for three days and then increase the dose to 150 mg twice a day. The doses should be taken at least eight hours apart. The second dose should not be taken close to bedtime. The drug is generally discontinued after twelve weeks.

Zyban and the patch have been used together to enhance quit rates. Side effects may include insomnia, dizziness, and dry mouth. Zyban is a prescription and should not be used in patients with a history of seizure, stroke, brain tumor, brain surgery or head injury, and eating disorders.

Interestingly, I had a coworker who made multiple attempts to quit her forty-year smoking habit. Despite serious heart and lung complications, she just couldn't quit. Recently, I was astonished to hear that she finally found a way to quit. She said, "Tell all of your patients about Zyban. Nothing had worked for me before. I finally found something that worked to help me quit!"

Varenicline (Chantix)[21]

While smoking, nicotine attaches to receptors within the brain and stimulates the release of dopamine, which produces a pleasurable sensation. Chantix attaches to these receptors instead and blocks the pleasurable chemicals. Dopamine is not released. If you smoke while taking Chantix, you don't get the positive payoffs. Smokers have stated that it doesn't taste the same and they don't enjoy smoking, which made it easier for them to quit.

This prescription medication is a powerful deterrent to smoking, but it does carry some troublesome side effects and should be used cautiously. The dose should begin one week before you set a quit date and adjusted to a therapeutic dose. In general, patients are treated for twelve weeks while smoking cessation behavioral strategies are implemented. You are reevaluated, and if you are doing well, you will be given the medication for another twelve weeks, then it is tapered down and discontinued.

One seventy-three-year-old smoker told me she had suffered from a second heart attack and was aware that smoking would eventually kill her. She tried everything to quit her pack a day habit. Finally, her cardiologist gave her a prescription of Chantix and it worked. "I smoked but nothing happened. It was like inhaling air. I didn't want to smoke anymore and I finally quit."

Depression and Suicide Thoughts

In addition to the nicotine withdrawal symptoms, there is a real perceived loss of an enjoyable habit. Some friendships centered around the habit of tobacco use and the social loss cause a great deal of anguish and distress. Many people who quit smoking will be anxious, irritable and have depressive thoughts. It is a side effect of nicotine withdrawal. Chantix can make these emotional and psychological symptoms worse. It is difficult to determine whether the negative mood is from Chantix or the act of quitting a tobacco habit. There have been some rare incidences of suicidal thoughts. According to the *Quick Reference Guide for Clinicians 2008 Update: Treating Tobacco Use and Dependence.*[20]

> Veranicline (Chantix) is an effective smoking cessation treatment that patients should be encouraged to use. See the Guideline and the FDA web site (www.fda.gov) for additional information on the safe and effective use of the medication. (31)

The following is a list of common Chantix considerations:[21]

- Watch carefully for psychological changes and report depressed mood, agitation, changes in behavior, and suicidal thoughts.
- Use cautiously if you have any kidney disease.
- Take with a full glass of water after eating.
- Avoid operating heavy equipment or machinery as the drug may cause drowsiness or dizziness.
- Alcohol makes the effects of Chantix much stronger.
- Do not stop Chantix suddenly; taper off instead.

In my experience, patients are fearful of using smoking cessation medications. Nicotine is highly addictive and many find it very difficult to quit. My recommendation is to contact one of the smoking experts listed at the end of this chapter. Talk with them about your particular habit. If you are a heavy user, I would definitely speak with your healthcare provider about these medications. However, many providers are not familiar with them. Educate yourself by speaking with a smoking expert and then be armed with your questions. In chapter 11, I share the things that you can do to have a stronger working relationship with your healthcare provider. Throw everything at this problem. There may be side effects from these medications, but nothing is worse than continued smoking! The next section of this chapter will contain behavior strategies that will help you become successful.

Behavior Strategies

There are a variety of behavior strategies that may be used along with medications to enhance your tobacco cessation efforts. First, there are common strategies that apply to all types of tobacco use and then specific ones for cigarette, cigar, and smokeless tobacco products. In the appendix, you will find a list of several smoking cessation strategies to help you quit.

Smokeless Tobacco (Quitting Tips)

Most of the smoking cessation tips will help you quit a smokeless tobacco habit with a few additional considerations.[22] A person who uses two cans a week of snuff gets as much nicotine as a 1½ pack a day smoker. Smokeless tobacco users are less common than cigarette and cigar users. Providing helpful quitting advice should come from experts experienced with this habit. I recommend that you contact one of the hotlines mentioned below to get the unique individualized help that you may need:

- National Cancer Institute's Smoking Cessation Quitline 1–877–448–7848
- National Network of Tobacco Cessation Quitlines 1–800 QUIT NOW or 1–800–784–8669

Some brands contain more nicotine than others. Switch to a brand with lower nicotine levels. The following list ranks them from highest to lowest amounts of nicotine:[22]

- Kodiak Wintergreen
- Skoal Longcut Straight
- Copenhagen Snuff
- Copenhagen Long Cut
- Skoal Bandits Mint
- Hawken Wintergreen

If you are unsure how addicted you have become to the nicotine in your smokeless tobacco, the following quiz may help you.

Smokeless Tobacco Addiction Quiz

Yes	No	I no longer get sick or dizzy when I dip or chew, like I did when I first started.
Yes	No	I dip more often and in different settings.
Yes	No	I've switched to stronger products, with more nicotine.
Yes	No	I swallow juice from my tobacco on a regular basis.
Yes	No	I sometimes sleep with dip or chew in my mouth.
Yes	No	I take my first dip or chew first thing in the morning.
Yes	No	I find it hard to go more than a few hours without dip or chew.
Yes	No	I have strong cravings when I go without dip or chew.
The more items you check, the more likely that you are addicted.		
*National Institute of Health		

The following list of reasons others gave for ending their smokeless tobacco habit was provided by the National Institute of Health. It may help you garner motivation to quit your tobacco habit.[22]

- Avoid health problems.
- I have sores in my mouth.
- I have bad breath and gum problems.
- My wife hates it.
- I want to be a good example for my children.
- Save money.
- My physician or dentist told me to quit.
- To prove I can do it.
- I don't want it to control my life anymore.

Tips for Quitting Smokeless Tobacco

Call a smokeless tobacco expert to talk about how you should quit.
Set a quit date.
Speak with your healthcare provider regarding whether the smoking cessation medications would help you with your smokeless tobacco habit.
Before your quit date, cut your use by half the amount.
Try a mint flavored substitute.
Try switching to a sugar free gum or lower nicotine product.
Cut back on when and where you chew or use snuff.
Wait 10 minutes before you satisfy a craving.
Pick 3 of your strongest triggers and stop using during those times.
Do not keep the tobacco in a place with easy access. Change the location.
*National Institute of Health

The first week is the roughest as you are coping with the same withdrawal symptoms as other tobacco users previously described. It won't be easy, but you can do it! Celebrate with your support team.

Take Away Points

You have learned that there are many nuances involved in a chronic tobacco habit. While your healthcare provider encourages you to quit, he or she is most likely not an expert in treating your tobacco addiction but rather a key member of your team. The staff that run reputable smoking hotlines or tobacco cessation counselors work with tobacco users every day. Call them. Let them walk you through the quitting process and meet your unique and individual needs. It's imperative that you quit not only for your own well-being but the health of your loved ones. Your children are watching you and mimicking your habits, the good as well as the bad. Your secondhand smoke is harming their health. There has never been a better time to quit than now.

> You gain strength, courage, and confidence by every experience in which you really stop to look fear in the face. You are able to say to yourself, "I have lived through this horror. I can take the next thing that comes along." You must do the thing, you think you cannot do.
>
> —Eleanor Roosevelt

Additional Information

National Cancer Institute (NCI): 1–800–4–CANCER or 1–800–422–6237

National Network of Tobacco Cessation Quitlines 1–800 QUIT NOW

American Cancer Society: 24 Hour Quitline 1–800–227–2345

For text support   http://smokefree.gov/

Quit Net www.quitnet.com

Nicotine Anonymous   www.nicotine-anonymous.org   1–877–879–6422

Centers for Disease Control and Prevention, Office On Smoking and Health   http://www.cdc.gov/tobacco/about/

American Lung Association www.lungusa.org 1–800–548–8252

American Heart Association   www.americanheart.org

Accredited Tobacco Treatment   Centers http://attudaccred.org/ programs

Mayo Clinic Residential Treatment Programs: www.mayoclinic. org/ndc/ or http://quit-smoking-advisor.com/05-Quit-Smoking-Programs/Residential/residential-quit-smoking-program-st-helena.html.

Those who think they have not time for bodily exercise
will sooner or later have to find time for illness.

—Edward Stanley, Earl of Derby,
in an address at Liverpool College, 1873

8

Physical Activity: Use It or Lose It

If you could bottle up exercise and place it into a pill, most chronic diseases would be eradicated, quality of life improved, and longevity prolonged. A sedentary, inactive life is a leading risk factor for a heart attack, stroke, cancer, diabetes, obesity, and many other debilitating diseases. Inactivity leads to premature aging, painful arthritis, hip fractures, and the need for earlier nursing home assistance due in part to the inability to pull oneself out of a chair.

While the benefits of physical activity are well-known, startling statistics indicate that very few actually do it. When asked, 52 percent of men and 46 percent of women reported that they regularly engaged in thirty minutes of moderate intensity exercise at least five days of the week.[1] Unfortunately, when wearing a device that actually detected movement, it was found that only 3.8 percent of men and 3.2 percent of women engaged in this level of physical activity.[1] Therefore, a myriad of health problems plague an inactive American population. Just a little bit of physical activity goes a long way in reducing these problems. The question remains, "If physical activity is so beneficial, why do so few people do it on a regular basis?" In this chapter, I review the rationale and importance for regular physical activity. More importantly, I walk you through simple realistic activities that you can implement to get you moving toward better health.

Energy Production

Our bodies are amazing creations. Every cell in the body needs energy to keep organs and tissues alive in order to function properly. Energy is made from the foods that you eat and the oxygen from the air. Recall from chapter 5 that food is digested and broken down into sugar that flows throughout your blood to all the cells and organs of the body. When it combines with oxygen, energy is made. Oxygen enters the lungs through the air that we breathe. The lungs contain a vast highway of arteries. Traveling along the highways are red blood cells that pick up the oxygen. The fresh oxygenated blood moves into the heart where it is pumped out to the rest of the body. The muscles throughout the body remove the oxygen from the blood cell and send it to tiny factories where the energy is made. Once the oxygen is removed, the blood cells return to the heart via the vein highways and are pumped back into the lungs to pick up more oxygen. While at rest, this process occurs 50 to 100 beats per minute throughout your life.

During an increase in physical activity, heart rate increases to supply greater amounts of oxygen to the exercising muscles. Three key body systems must work well together to be able to deliver oxygen to the working muscles: lungs, heart, and muscles. The lungs must be able to expand deeply to exchange oxygen. The heart must remain strong, pumping blood into healthy, open highways. The muscles must be able to extract the oxygen as the blood passes by and have enough factories to make energy.

Physical activity strengthens all of these systems. Additional benefits include increased muscle strength, prolonged endurance, and in most cases, a psychological sense of well-being.

Anaerobic versus Aerobic Energy Production

We have two systems that make energy. One is called the "aerobic" system, which uses oxygen, and the other is the "anaerobic" system that does not need oxygen to make energy. If you needed to run out of a burning building or away from an attacking grizzly bear, you would need a very rapid energy supply. You couldn't wait for several minutes while your heart and respiratory rate increased to deliver extra oxygen into your muscles. You need to run now! The anaerobic system provides a burst of energy, but it only lasts a minute or two, just long enough for the aerobic system to kick in. Sprinters train to strengthen their anaerobic system.

The aerobic system is responsible for most of our energy needs, but it takes a few minutes to kick in. As previously described, the food that you eat is eventually broken down into sugar or stored as fat. When sugar combines with oxygen, aerobic energy is made. This energy system is called aerobic because it needs oxygen to make energy. In highly fit people, aerobic energy can last for a very long time. Marathon runners train to strengthen their aerobic system.

As physical work increases, a great deal of blood is shunted or moves away from your core organs out to the exercising muscles to meet the demands for more oxygen. The heart and respiratory rate increase dramatically to help speed up energy production. These changes are uncomfortable for sedentary people who aren't used to exercise. It takes a few minutes for the body to adjust to the work demands. I think many people hate exercise in part because of the uncomfortable first few minutes of exercise while waiting for the aerobic system to kick in. This discomfort leads to a great deal of misunderstanding.

Another way to think of this barrier is with a lake example. Think back to the last time that you jumped into a cold lake. It was probably a hot summer day and you wanted to cool off. Your blood was close to the skin to help cool you. When you suddenly jumped into the cold lake, the blood immediately began to move back to your core vital organs to keep them warm. You actually felt pain and discomfort for a few minutes while your body adjusted to the dramatic change in body temperature. Your blood supply was readjusting. However, after a few minutes, an amazing thing happened. Your body temperature acclimated and you could float in the cold water for an hour and no longer notice the lake temperature. That initial movement of blood was uncomfortable, but eventually, those sensations went away and the experience was pleasant. The same type of thing happens in exercise. The blood supply needs to move out of the core organs into the exercising muscles of your body. That movement is uncomfortable for the first few minutes. Once the blood is in the muscles and the aerobic system kicks in, the discomfort goes away for most people.

Another misconception is that you have to work really hard to get any benefit from the physical activity. In fact, any movement helps. Strenuous exercise is uncomfortable and can cause injuries. Later in this chapter, I will teach you how to track your heart rate and keep it at a comfortable pace so that you can begin to enjoy the exercise experience. Understanding what is happening to your body is the first step in being more physically active.

Benefits of Physical Activity

In simplest terms, "fitness" is defined as the ability to have enough energy to feel good while doing the activities of daily living. A more professional definition was provided by fitness expert James Skinner:[2]

Muscles involved in exercise produce a significant amount of energy by combining foodstuffs with oxygen...Your ability to engage in sustained high levels of physical activity without significant fatigue is determined by your body's ability to deliver oxygenated blood to your muscles, and the ability of your muscles to extract the oxygen from the blood and utilize it for the production of energy... (57)

An unconditioned person will not be able to make as much energy as the fit person and will tire quickly with minimal activity. A fit person has an amazing ability to do more work with minimal effort because his or her body is so much stronger and efficient. Even people with serious medical conditions can improve their ability to make energy. Daily activities such as mowing the lawn, carrying groceries, or lifting a small child will be much easier to do without fatigue.

Health Benefits of Physical Activity

Heart Disease	Strengthens the heart muscle, widens coronary arteries around the heart and develops extra arteries.
Cancers	Improves the removal of toxins.
Diabetes	Burns excess blood sugar.
Lung Diseases	Lungs are able to inhale and exhale more efficiently.
Obesity	Burns triglycerides and stored fat.
High Blood Pressure	Widens arteries, which lowers blood pressure and the need for medication.
Abnormal Cholesterol	Helps to raise HDL (good) cholesterol, slightly lowers LDL (bad) cholesterol and VLDL (very bad) cholesterol.
Arthritis	Strengthens muscles around joints and reduces pain.
Bones	Enhances calcium absorption and improves balance to prevent falls.
Muscles	Extracts more oxygen and makes more energy.
Insomnia	Improves sleep.
Stress	Burns adrenalin to reduce annoying stress hormones.
Poor Self Image/ Depression	Improves self-image. Produces "feel good" endorphin chemicals released with exercise.

Intensity of Physical Activity

Physical activity can be defined as any action that gets you moving. It may vary from a simple ten-minute walk in your neighborhood to running several miles on a treadmill. You may have the misunderstanding that only certain types of exercise are beneficial. This is a common misconception that many people believe, "If I'm not in a gym working out vigorously, my activity doesn't count. I'm a failure, so why bother." It's an "all or nothing" mentality. This thinking is not only inaccurate; it's dangerous. A sedentary lifestyle profoundly increases risk for a heart attack and stroke. We were created to move. The important point to capture here is that even small improvements are a victory and a positive step toward a healthier life. I hope that throughout this chapter, you begin to think differently about simple realistic physical activities that you can add to your daily life. Walking can be initiated by most people and results in major health benefits.

Medical Clearance before Physical Activity

Before you begin any exercise program or physical activity, you need to be sure that you are healthy enough to participate. It is a good idea to get a physical and seek medical clearance if you have any type of heart condition or other serious medical problem, have experienced any chest discomfort with activity or at rest, dizziness episodes, bone or joint problems, if you are taking medication for high blood pressure, or have any other reason why you feel you might become harmed during exercise.[3]

Current Recommendations

While all activity counts, it is also important that you understand what constitutes an optimal exercise program. Current 2013 lifestyle recommendations for physical activity advise that individuals should have forty minutes of moderate to vigorous aerobic activity three to four times a week.[4]

> Most health benefits occur with at least 150 minutes (2 hours and 30 minutes) a week of moderate intensity physical activity, such as brisk walking. Additional benefits occur with more physical activity…Some physical activity is better than none…For most health outcomes, additional benefits occur as the amount of physical activity increases through higher intensity, greater frequency, and at longer duration. (30)

The ideal program consists of a five-minute warm-up before thirty to forty minutes of aerobic exercise, followed by some light to moderate weight lifting and a five-minute cooldown. Most healthcare providers recommend this type of program, as it provides the best medical improvements in health. However, it may be too unrealistic for many people to follow who may become easily overwhelmed and discouraged. I wanted you to be aware of what the recent guidelines recommend. In this chapter, I will describe simpler ways to get moving that you may feel more confident to initiate and sustain.

Importance of Warm-Up and Cooldowns

Warm-Up

A warm-up prior to exercise is important because it jumpstarts your aerobic energy production. Your heart and respiratory rate increase, blood moves from your core organs to your exercising muscles and aerobic energy production kicks in. Stretching should be a part of your warm-up because it will prevent muscle, tendon, and joint injury. Any activity can serve as the warm-up. If you are walking, just begin at a slower, more relaxed pace and increase your speed by the end of five minutes.

Cooldown

Immediately after exercise, the majority of the blood supply is being pumped to your muscles. Blood needs to move back to your core organs. Your blood pressure and heart rate need to return to normal. The cooldown will allow this process to happen. If you suddenly stop exercising without a cooldown, the blood will pool in your lower legs. You may feel dizzy, nauseated, and could develop an abnormal heart rhythm. Decreasing the intensity of your activity works well for the cooldown. As an example, if you were walking at a faster pace, decrease your speed. Warm-ups and cooldowns include continuous exercise but at a much lower level of intensity.

Aerobic Exercise

Ideally, once your body has warmed up, a good aerobic workout is at least thirty minutes of sustained activity. If you are not conditioned or unfit, your aerobic exercise should be significantly less. For some people, it may be only five or ten minutes of aerobic work. You need to begin slowly. I advise my patients that anything physically active will be beneficial so just get started doing something. Conditioning occurs as your body responds to the increased workload or physical demands of your activity. Your exercise should slightly stress the body; however, this activity should not be so strenuous or painful that it forces you to quit. I recommend two methods to ensure that your workout is not too strenuous: Target Heart Rate and Talk Test.

Target Heart Rate

The target heart rate range indicates the level of your heart rate or pulse for aerobic conditioning during exercise. The low number represents the lowest workout intensity. The highest number indicates the highest level of workout intensity during your exercise. You should monitor your pulse and work within the two numbers. If you take your pulse and it is too slow, you increase your exercise intensity. If you take your pulse and it is too fast, you should reduce your exercise intensity. According to the American College of Sport's Medicine, the goal for most aerobic exercise is to work between 40 percent to 85 percent of your maximum heart rate (MHR) depending upon your level of fitness.[5] The MHR is the fastest rate that your heart will beat for your age. It varies from person to person and becomes lower with age. People who are less fit should begin working within the lowest target heart rate ranges and those who are in excellent condition may choose to work within the higher ranges.

Target Heart Rate Zone[6]

Age	Target Heart Rate Zone 50% to 85%	Average Maximum Heart Rate, 100%
20 years	100 to 170 beats per minute	200 beats per minute
30 years	95 to 162 beats per minute	190 beats per minute
35 years	93 to 157 beats per minute	185 beats per minute
40 years	90 to 153 beats per minute	180 beats per minute
45 years	88 to 149 beats per minute	175 beats per minute
50 years	85 to 145 beats per minute	170 beats per minute
55 years	83 to 140 beats per minute	165 beats per minute
60 years	80 to 136 beats per minute	160 beats per minute
65 years	78 to 132 beats per minute	155 beats per minute
70 years	75 to 128 beats per minute	150 beats per minute
Check with your healthcare provider about your rates, which may be different if you are taking certain medications such as beta-blockers.		
*American Heart Association		

Your target heart rate may also be calculated. You may view the calculation in the appendix. You will be asked to determine your maximum heat rate (MHR), which is 220 minus your age. However, the most accurate way to know how fast your heart will beat or your MHR is with a stress treadmill test. Your heart rate is measured during exercising and the maximum or peak rate is recorded. The exercise staff at your local gym can also calculate your target heart rates.

You can wear a heart rate monitor or take your pulse to determine your heart rate during exercise. To take your pulse, first, place your index and middle fingers gently over your carotid artery in your neck just under your jaw bone. Apply gentle light pressure until you feel your pulse. You can also place your fingers over the boney prominence in your wrist. Count your pulse for 10 seconds and multiple it by 6 to calculate your heart rate per minute. While you can practice taking your pulse, I recommend that you purchase a device that measures your pulse. The technology is rapidly exploding and there are many devices, which monitor pulse rate easily and accurately.

Talk Test[7]

The "talk test" is a simple method to determine if you are working too hard. It works best if you use it while walking. You should be able to carry on a conversation without feeling too winded or short of breath to speak during the activity. You would find singing too hard to do. Activities of vigorous intensity would cause you to pause in order to take a breath in between a few words. If you are having a difficult time talking, decrease your intensity.

Key Points

If you are taking certain blood pressure medications such as beta-blockers, your maximum heart rate will automatically be lower. Most beta-blockers work by blocking the ability of the heart rate to increase under mental or physical stress and lower resting heart rates. You should speak with your healthcare provider or a fitness specialist to help you determine an appropriate target heart rate if you are taking these types of medications. If you have not exercised in a very long time and you are terribly out of shape, I would begin with your intensity at a low number of 40 percent off your maximum heart rate. Check with your healthcare provider before you initiate any strenuous physical activity.

Types of Aerobic Activity

The perfect aerobic activity reaches an intensity where your skin begins to glisten and you break a slight sweat. Brisk walking, biking, tennis, dancing, yard work, swimming, water aerobics, and Jazzercize (movement to music) are examples of moderate aerobic activity. The key is to engage in activities that are fun! The following table indicates how many calories you burn with various aerobic activities. It provides you with an idea of which activities involve a greater intensity of work.

Calories Burned Per Minute of Physical Activity[8]

Moderate Physical Activity	Approximate Calories/hour 154 pound person
Hiking	370
Light gardening/yard work	330
Dancing	330
Golfing (walking and carrying clubs)	330
Bicycling (less than 10 mph)	290
Walking (3.5 mph)	280
Weight lifting (general light workout)	220
Stretching	180
Vigorous Physical Activity	**Approximate Calories/hour 154 pound person**
Running/jogging (5 mph)	590
Bicycling (greater than 10 mph)	590
Swimming (slow freestyle laps)	510
Doing aerobics	480
Walking (4.5 mph)	460
Heavy yard work (chopping wood)	440
Weight lifting (vigorous effort)	440
Playing basketball (vigorous)	440

Calories burned per hour will be higher for persons who weigh more than 154 pounds and lower for persons who weigh less.

*Preventive Cardiovascular Nurses Association
National Guidelines and Tools, 2009
*Adapted from US Department of Agriculture
Dietary Guidelines for Americans, 2005

Weight or Strength Training

A great strategy for weight control is to add resistance training or light weight lifting to your exercise routine a few times per week. If you have more muscle, your body will have a higher metabolism. You will literally burn more calories while sitting in a chair if you have more muscle mass. Secondly, stronger muscles maintain proper body alignment, which protects you from potential injury. My husband suffered a serious knee injury in college. The damage was so severe that he now has "bone on bone" arthritis. However, because he regularly exercises the muscles that support his knee, he has developed a natural splint. If he accidentally twists or turns his knee, it is protected from additional injury. Finally, increased muscle mass improves body image as well. You look and feel better. The figure below shows how muscle changes with simple resistance training or light weight lifting. Fat is burned for energy and shrinks while muscle mass increases. When you build muscle through resistance training or weight lifting, you also burn fat for fuel. You end up with more muscle and less fat.

Effect of Light Weight Lifting on Fat and Muscle

Out of Shape

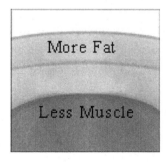

Excellent Condition

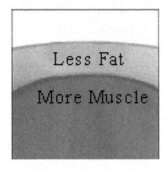

It is safer to begin with lighter weights and more frequent repetitions. Lifting weights after aerobic exercise is better since your muscles are already warmed up. Simple weight lifting strategies at home involve:

- Using your arms to do pushups off of your kitchen table.
- Standing up and sitting down from a chair.
- Standing by a chair or table and balancing on one leg at a time.
- Lifting a soup can ten times for three repetitions.
- Walking up and down a hill.
- Taking the stairs whenever possible.

A professional exercise trainer or resistance training class is another option to get you started. Be creative and have fun with the activity.

Potential Problems While Engaging in Physical Activity

Unusual Pain or Discomfort

In the 1980s, Jane Fonda led a fitness craze that was captured by the phrase, "Go for the burn." She advocated working hard and not being afraid of vigorous exercise. "No pain, no gain." However, many injuries occurred from this intense approach to exercise. If you develop pain or discomfort while exercising, it is important that you stop immediately and seek medical assistance. Even if you experience the symptoms for one hour following exercise, you should immediately call your healthcare provider. Heart attack and stroke symptoms are the most dangerous.

Warning Signs of a Heart Attack[9]

Heart Attack Warning Signs
Burning, heaviness, pressure, tightness or squeezing sensation in chest.
Discomfort in jaw, shoulder, back, between the shoulder blades or down the arm.
Shortness of breath.
Fatigue, lightheadedness or weakness.
Nausea, indigestion, fatigue.
*American Heart Association

FAST Stroke Warning Signs[10]

(FAST) Stroke Warning Signs
Face Drooping: Does one side of the face droop or is it numb? Ask the person to smile. Is the person's smile uneven?
Arm Weakness: Is one arm weak or numb? Ask the person to raise both arms. Does one arm drift downward?
Speech Difficulty: Is speech slurred? Is the person unable to speak or hard to understand? Ask the person to repeat a simple sentence like, "The sky is blue." Is the sentence repeated correctly?
Time to call 911: If someone shows any of these symptoms, even if the symptoms go away, call 911 and get the person to the hospital immediately. Check the time so you'll know when the first symptoms appeared.
*American Stroke Association

Physical Activity on Hot Days

Muscle contractions during physical activity produce heat and warm the body. Sweating and evaporation help to cool the body to protect the core organs. However, if the outside temperature is very warm, it will be harder to cool the body and temperature will rise. The Heat Index may be obtained from the National Weather Service and shows the cumulative effect of hotter temperatures and humidity.[11] You may view the Heat Index table in the appendix. As the heat and temperature increase, so does your risk for heat stroke. Use caution when exercising during hot temperatures.

Heat Exhaustion

Exercising in very hot humid conditions is the leading cause of heat exhaustion. When exercising in the heat, the heart rate and sweating increase more rapidly to cool the body. Dehydration, secondary to sweating, may quickly lead to a dangerous rise in core body temperature. The very young and the very old are most vulnerable, but anyone can be stricken with this disease. Certain medical conditions may increase your vulnerability. Dehydration occurs more readily if you are taking high blood pressure medication. Obese persons or those with heart and lung disease will have more difficulty cooling their body.

Early symptoms of trouble may include: heavy sweating, fatigue, excess thirst, nausea, lightheadedness, and feeling faint. Stopping the physical activity, increasing fluid intake, and cooling the body will correct the disorder. Working within your target heat rate will help avoid this complication. Your heart rate will rise much more quickly during hot climates forcing you to back off your intensity. Generally, it is recommended to "drink 2 cups of fluid 2 hours before exercise, and drink during exercise at a rate that matches sweat losses." (303)[5]

Heat Stroke

If heat exhaustion is untreated, it may progress to heatstroke. Body temperatures over 105°F or higher are diagnostic of heat stroke.[12] This is a medical emergency! The body needs cooled immediately to avoid damage to vital organs and death. Chicago, Illinois, experienced dangerous hot temperatures in 1995 that resulted in 485 heat-related deaths. Across the nation, over 8,000 heat-related deaths occurred between 1979 to 1999.[13] Check with your healthcare provider about your risk for this problem. Caution must be used if you decide to exercise during extreme hot weather. Follow the Heat Index guidelines and avoid exercise outdoors in the heat on dangerous days. The following tips may help:

- Work out within an air-conditioned building.
- Reduce your exercise intensity.

- Exercise during the cooler times of the day: early morning or late evening.
- Wear lightweight clothing.
- Maintain fluids.

Engaging in physical activity during hot climates has the potential to lead to very dangerous heat-related complications. Use caution.

Physical Activity on Cold Days

When the weather is very cold, the body has to work much harder to maintain body temperature. Arteries constrict or tighten, which limits the amount of oxygen flowing through them. Shoveling heavy wet snow requires a great deal of energy, muscle, and work. Your heart rate and blood pressure dramatically increase. If you have any type of underlying heart disease, the strain may induce a heart attack. Speak with your healthcare provider about your risk. Wear several layers of clothing when you are out in the cold. A great deal of heat is lost through the head so wear a hat. Cover your hands to stay warm and avoid frostbite. Be especially mindful of cold temperatures on windy days when the wind chill increases your risk for frostbite. You may view a copy of the Cold Wind Chill Index in the appendix.

Physical Activity at Higher Altitudes[5]

At higher altitudes, less oxygen is available. The heart rate and blood pressure may increase to dangerous levels in order to deliver adequate oxygen to the tissues. The lower oxygen content could result in a heart attack or stroke. Acute mountain sickness begins about 6 to 12 hours after rising over 8,000 feet. Symptoms include headache, fatigue, nausea, vomiting, and sleep disturbances, which may abate after 3 to 7 days or a descent to a lower altitude. High altitude pulmonary edema is swelling that occurs within the lungs and is a life-threatening condition. Symptoms include very rapid breathing, increased heart rate, shortness of breath, pink frothy congested cough, and blue-colored skin due to very low oxygen levels within the blood. High altitude cerebral edema is swelling that occurs within the brain and is another life-threatening problem. Symptoms include severe weakness, staggering gait, ashen gray skin color, drowsiness, confusion, and coma. If you experience any of these symptoms, you should call 911 immediately!

Exercise exacerbates the challenges at high altitudes. The following recommendations reduce your risk for experiencing high altitude complications:[5]

- Ascend slowly.
- Climb in stages. If traveling higher than 10,000 feet, limit your climb rate to 1,000 feet per day.
- Drink plenty of fluids to avoid dehydration.
- Avoid overexertion and hypothermia.
- Eat a high carbohydrate diet to reduce symptoms.
- Ask your doctor for a prescription of some medications that may prevent altitude problems.
- Use your target heart rate to guide your activities. It will speed up when oxygen levels are too low. Reduce the intensity of your activities.

Generally altitudes below 5,000 feet are not a problem.[5] For most people, acclamation to the higher altitudes occurs after three days. When I travel to Denver to visit relatives, I give myself a day or two to adjust to the altitude before I initiate exercise. While I'm a little bit more short of breath, I tolerate the altitude well. However, I did suffer from acute mountain sickness when we rented a condo that was at 11,000 feet in Breckenridge, Colorado. Nausea, a splitting headache, fatigue, and blue-colored nail beds remained until we descended. Higher altitudes can really impact your ability to exercise so use caution.

Physical Activity and Pollution

Emerging research indicates that pollution may increase your risk for a heart attack and stroke. The American Heart Association recommends that people with underlying cardiac conditions or lung problems avoid exercise in areas of high traffic.[14] It would be safer to exercise in parks or at times during the day when pollution levels are lower. The Air Quality Index may also provide information when you should avoid pollution and exercise indoors.[15] You may view a copy of the Air Quality Index in the appendix.

Other Considerations

Physical Activity and Excess Weight

Approximately 70 percent of Americans are either overweight or obese.[1] Starting an exercise program can be both intimidating and embarrassing. Water aerobics is a wonderful way to start, but it can be terribly uncomfortable putting on a bathing suit and entering a crowded pool. Just know that you aren't alone. Another great idea is to start with short walks. Monitor your target heart rate to guide your speed. Each small step is a victory.

Physical Activity and Aging

After age 30, inactive people lose 3 percent to 5 percent of muscle mass every ten years with a total loss of 15 percent by age 60.[16] Muscle loss decreases metabolism, which can lead to weight gain. Joints become stiffer. Flexibility and balance are also reduced. Falls become more likely and seniors become more fragile. Half of seniors whose fall requires hospitalization will not be alive one year after the event.[12] Physical activity improves balance, which reduces falls. Lightweight lifting strengthens the body and counters much of the muscle loss due to the aging process. Therefore, in order to avoid a broken hip and nursing home, seniors must begin to think differently about physical activity. The goal of life is to age gracefully. How those final chapters are spent depends in great part upon the mental and physical fitness of the body. Exercise not only improves the quantity of life, but also the quality of those years.

Increasing Physical Activity Throughout Your Day

So far, I have talked about implementing the best type of exercise program safely. This activity involves a five-minute warm-up, twenty to thirty minutes of aerobic activity in your target heart rate zone, followed by some light weight lifting, ending with a five-minute cooldown. The experts admonish all of us to do this physical activity on most days of the week.[1] However, statistics show that few of us perform this level of intensity. We have become far too sedentary, but we haven't always been this way.

Researchers compared the household management (HM) activities of women between the ages of nineteen and sixty-four years old from data obtained in 1965 and 2010.[17] The activities included time spent in food preparation, dish washing, laundry, and general housework. On average, the women in 1965 were more active and spent 27.7 hours per week performing these activities while women in 2010 spent only 13.3 hours per week. Modern appliances may have played some role in the decrease in activity levels. In 1970, less than 1 percent of all families owned a microwave, but by 2005, 90 percent owned one. In 1970, less than 20 percent of households had a dishwasher, but by 2005, over 60 percent of all families had a dishwasher. During this time period, caloric expenditure decreased in nonworking women by 42 percent and working women by 30 percent, while time spent in watching media increased 8.3 hours per week. No doubt that technology played some role in this lower activity level that was observed.

One of the first studies to examine active employment versus inactive employment involved men in England.[18] Between 1949 and 1950, 31,000 male transport workers between the ages of thirty-five to sixty-five years old were studied. Double-decker bus drivers climbed on average between 500 to 750 steps a day for their job while taxi drivers sat 90 percent of their time. The researchers found a 20 percent higher rate of "sudden death" among the less active workers. At first, the medical community did not believe that physical activity could play such a pivotal role in health. However, similar results were found in a study of 110,000 active postal workers compared to sedentary civil servants and 3,263 active longshoreman (cargo handlers). Physical activity was found to be protective.

In fact, research has supported that all physical activity counts.[5] In the final section, I describe simple realistic physical activities that you can incorporate into your daily life in order to reduce your risk for a heart attack and stroke.

Walk a Dog Even If You Don't Have One

Really...

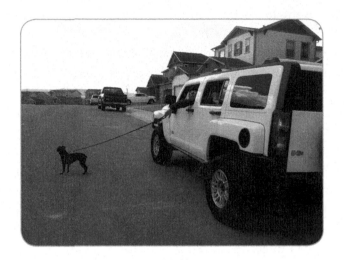

Much Better...

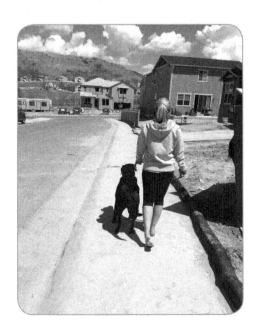

Walking

Walking can be done by everyone. If you are really out of shape, just start with a walk five minutes from your house and then come back. Do that for a week or two, and if you are tolerating the activity well, increase it by five minutes. Walk in the cool of the evening or earlier in the morning. Take your spouse or a friend to have an accountability partner. If you are having a lazy day, the other person will help motivate you to get moving and vice versa. It's a great way to unwind and share the concerns of the day. Listen to music or a book on tape. Wear comfortable shoes and layered clothing. Don't forget your sunscreen, a hat, and sunglasses. Try and walk on a flat surface if the activity is new for you.

Adjust your intensity according to your "target heart rate" or "talk test" previously described. You should be able to carry on a conversation without getting too short of breath. Many people use a pedometer. This device is attached to your belt and senses leg movement. It counts each step. The ultimate goal is to walk 10,000 steps each day.[19] You can start slow and increase the number of steps each week until you reach your goal. Many people wear the pedometer while at work. If they fall short of their goal of a certain number of steps in a day, they add a walk once home. You can purchase a pedometer from most sports stores and new styles of pedometers are being developed. If you have a smart phone, check with your carrier for some of the new apps that monitor your steps while you carry the phone. You can also accumulate ten-minute walks three different times throughout your day to reach your physical activity goal. Bouts of moderate activity have been shown to be beneficial and count as your daily exercise.[19] The following list may help you consider other ways to incorporate physical activity into your daily life. Be creative and find fun things to do. Remember, that even small physical activity counts!

Activities throughout the Day

- Park your car further away.
- Take an activity break.
- Go for a walk at lunch.
- Take the stairs whenever you can.
- Do your housework at a brisk pace.
- Go dancing instead of a movie.
- Try water aerobics.
- Go bowling.
- Golf but walk, do not ride in a cart.
- Play with your children or grandchildren.
- Take them for a nature walk.
- Play catch with them.
- Go for a walk after dinner.

Becoming a Habit

Whenever you begin any new behavior, it takes a few weeks for it to become routine that you don't even have to think about it anymore. Increasing your physical activity is no exception. As an example, I worked in a heart institute where our offices were on the second floor, but we counseled patients on the first floor. We carried beepers and were notified whenever it was time to see a patient. The elevator was next to our office and too convenient to use it to go up and down one floor. I had to go out of the way to use the stairs. However, I knew that using the stairs would give me some exercise and would be good for my blood pressure. For the first few weeks, I had to intentionally think about going the longer route to access the stairs. After a few weeks, my brain learned the new route and my body automatically moved to the stairs. A new behavior becomes a habit when you don't have to think about doing it anymore. *Incognito: The Secret Lives of the Brain* was written by a neuroscientist, David Eagleman, who explores the unconscious influences of the brain on our behaviors.[20] I highly recommend this book to help you gain greater insight into the role that the brain plays in learning healthier habits.

Personal Story

Finding time to incorporate physical activity into an already busy schedule is challenging for all of us. Sweaty hair and boring exercise were certainly major barriers for me as well. Those first few uncomfortable minutes were enough to halt the best of my exercise intentions. However, when I hit the midlife years, my blood pressure and cholesterol went through the roof, forcing me to reconsider my inactive lifestyle. Faced with a choice of increasing the medications or taking my own advice and starting an exercise program, I decided to get moving.

A friend invited me to a Jazzercize class where I finally found an activity that was fun to do. It was movement to music, almost like dancing. I saw women of various ages and sizes with sculpted bodies moving to the music. The hour was divided into aerobic work followed by light weight lifting, which I was able to do. I couldn't do all of the steps of course, but as long as I kept moving, it didn't seem to matter. After a few weeks, the exercise started to feel good. My joints felt like they were lubricated, the weight was coming down, and I saw muscle definition that I didn't know I had.

I'm still exercising, but I do different things. Sometimes, it's an aerobics class while other times, it's a quiet walk in the woods. The secret to physical activity for me was finding things that I "love" to do and viewing exercise differently. Frankly, I want to avoid a stroke and a nursing home for as long as I possibly can. I no longer view exercise or physical activity as a burden, but rather an activity that buys me time for a longer, better quality of life. I would like you to begin to think differently about what you would like to do as well. What activities did you enjoy as a child or teen? Where might you be able to sneak some physical activity into your life?

Take Away Points

Adding physical activity to a sedentary life is challenging because most Americans spend a great deal of their day sitting on a chair in front of a computer or television screen. We've grown accustomed to inactivity. However, headlines are beginning to emerge that "sitting is the new smoking."[21] Our inactivity is killing us. Research has shown that all activity counts to help counter the damage.[4] Even getting up out of the chair and walking a bit every hour is helpful.[21] Small amounts of activity are better than no activity. As you consider your risk for a heart attack and stroke, think of simple ways that you can incorporate physical activity into your daily life. Make it fun and be realistic. Each step is a victory toward better health. Remember, a little bit of physical activity goes a very long way, so get moving. Use it or you will most certainly lose it.

God grant me the serenity to accept the things I cannot change;
The courage to change the things I can;
And the wisdom to know the difference.

—Serenity Prayer by Theologian, Reinhold Niebuhr

9

Controlling Your Response to Life's Stressors

Stress is an unavoidable part of everyone's life. It comes from a variety of places and situations. Sometimes, the triggers are small, such as spilling a cup of milk or dramatic like the death of a loved one. The responses may range from simple annoyance to a cataclysmic explosion of anger and hostility. Your risk for a heart attack and stroke becomes much greater, depending upon your stress response. In an attempt to lift the negative mood induced by stress, an individual may engage in behaviors that are harmful to health, such as smoking, overeating, alcohol abuse, and sedentary activities.[1]

The harmful behaviors increase the "feel good" endorphins produced in the brain, but the relief is only temporary. It comes at a very high price. Smoking causes a great deal of trauma to the linings of the arteries. Consuming junk foods high in sugar, salt, and fat result in excess weight. High blood pressure, abnormal cholesterol levels, and increased risk for diabetes follows. Sitting for prolonged periods of time distracting oneself with television or a computer screen makes everything worse. These escape behaviors provide only temporary relief from the stressors of everyday life. Yet individuals engage in a myriad of harmful behaviors in an attempt to improve their emotions. In this chapter, I explore how stress harms the body and I provide you with alternative coping skills that you may consider for a healthier more positive approach to the stressful events in your life.

Stress

Stress is defined as your body's response to any psychological, emotional, or physical demand placed upon it. Fear, anger, anxiety, worry, etc., are the usual psychological responses, but stress is not always negative. It can be good, such as having a new baby, celebrating a wedding, or spending time with relatives over the holidays. It can be bad due to the exhaustion from caring for a new baby, fretting over the endless details of wedding planning or the arguments that often ensue with contentious relatives during holiday gatherings. Your body is unable to tell the difference between positive and negative stress. However, individuals recover faster from positive stressors with minimal damage to the body compared to negative stressors.

When the stress response is activated, the body responds immediately. Your brain is getting you ready to take some type of action. In the 1930s, physiologist Walter Cannon was the first to describe this phenomenon as the "fight or flight response."[2] When faced with an immediate stress or threat from a grizzly bear attack or a burning building, the body releases a powerful chemical called adrenalin. This chemical immediately causes an increase in your heart rate, breathing, blood pressure, blood sugar, and oxygen level to increase energy production to your muscles. Interestingly, adrenalin causes your gastrointestinal system to temporarily shut down. All energy is conserved for the "fight or flight response." Adrenalin is the chemical that helps you to move or act quickly. While this response is needed to escape the danger, it can be deadly if activated too frequently.

Hans Seyle described three stages individuals move through when faced with prolonged stressful situations: Alarm Stage, Adaptation Stage, and Stage of Exhaustion.[3] During the Alarm Stage, the "fight or flight response" is activated by an adrenalin surge. In the Adaptation Stage, the body adjusts to the ongoing stressor. In the Stage of Exhaustion, the constant bombardment of adrenalin damages all of the arteries throughout the body and increases risk for many disorders. It is imperative to cope well with the stressors of your life, to shut off the adrenalin surging through your body.

Harm to the Body

Adrenalin causes the blood to coagulate faster to stop any bleeding if you are injured during the "fight or flight response." However, the stickier blood, higher heart rate, blood pressure, and blood sugar are hard on the arteries and increase your risk for a heart attack and stroke.[1] Protracted stress reduces the ability of the body to fight infection as well.[1] Most frightening is the link between chronic stress and cancer.[4]

Personal Story

While in graduate school, I worked as a research assistant within a National Institute of Health (NIH) sponsored study titled, "Effect of Mindfulness Based Stress Reduction on Immune Function, Quality of Life and Coping in Women Newly Diagnosed with Early Stage Breast Cancer."[4] Primarily, they wanted to examine how stress alters immunity in women diagnosed with very early stage breast cancer.

In the study, half of the women were given eight weeks of meditation therapy based on the Jon Kabat-Zinn book titled *Full Catastrophe Living*. Topics taught within the 2.5 hour sessions included: breath awareness, sitting, walking, meditation, and yoga. The control group did not receive the intervention. Psychological surveys were administered to evaluate perceived stress levels along with other variables. Saliva samples were obtained to measure cortisol levels, which are elevated during times of stress. When cortisol levels are higher, the number of natural killer cells that circulate in the blood are lower.[5] Natural killer cells recognize the harmful cancer cell and produce a chemical called a cytokine, which destroys the cancer. Blood tests were drawn to measure the number of natural killer cells and cytokines present within the women. The researchers were testing whether the meditation intervention would lower perceived stress and cortisol levels and thereby enhance the number of natural killer cells and cytokines available to fight the breast cancer.

Upon completion of the study, the women who received the meditation therapy had lower levels of cortisol and a greater number of the natural killer cells and cytokines compared to the women who did not receive the therapy.[4] The meditation therapy appeared to strengthen their immunity and ability to fight cancer better than the control group. Dr. Janusek, the team leader, believes that one day, stress reduction techniques will be prescribed along with other cancer treatments to boost immunity. While this research is still emerging, it spoke volumes about the importance of managing daily stress, not only for heart attack and stroke prevention but cancer as well.

Stressors

Many individuals deny that the stress in their life is a problem. When working with patients, I generally say, "If you think that you have too much stress in your life, you probably do." Perceived stress is very subjective. What one person may find stressful, another may find delightful. As an example, I find yard work stressful, while my husband loves to dig holes in the ground and stir up dirt. I love to engage an audience with motivational stories that improve health while someone else is paralyzed with terrible stage fright. The point is that perceived stress is as individual as our DNA.

Daily stress comes at us from many different places, circumstances, and situations. Work-related stressful scenarios are challenging because individuals often feel powerless to do anything about it. They are trapped within what I call a "toxic work environment" with no escape from the situation. It takes a great deal of courage to confront the problems head on with a "fight response" or to change jobs with a "flight response." Either approach is stressful, but doing nothing may be even more harmful to your health. A book that I found very helpful is a new release by "CEO Whisperer," Debra Benton titled, The *CEO Difference: How to Climb, Crawl, and Leap Your Way to the Next Level of Your Career.* The author provides excellent tips on how to get along and succeed within the corporate world, but her tips are useful for everyone in any work environment. It will help to lower your stress if you can learn how to handle challenging situations and difficult people.

Challenging personal relationships cause a great deal of stress. Researchers asked 150 older couples to discuss a "sore subject" for six minutes."[6] The conversations were scored based on their levels of hostility. Coronary artery calcium (CAC) heart scans were obtained to measure levels of heart disease. Refer to chapter 2 for information on this test. Comparisons were made between the levels of hostility and heart disease. In the relationships where the husbands were verbally hostile and the wives were controlling, CAC scores or heart disease was significantly higher. In another study, approximately 9,000 mostly married British civil servants were followed for twelve years.[7] Again, the researchers found that those within the "worst relationships" had 34 percent more heart attacks than those within "good relationships." Stressful personal relationships increase risk for heart disease. What is the best course of action for these difficult situations? It isn't always easy to know what to do. I recommend that you try professional counseling to resolve some of the conflict. However, far too many people do nothing and remain in toxic environments paying the price with adverse health.

Other events are so out of our control that they overwhelm the most calm among us. Following the aftermath of Hurricane Katrina there was a doubling of heart attacks.[8] Initially, the first week after the 2011 Japanese Fukushima earthquake, there were 70 percent more cardiac arrests.[9] The numbers kept diminishing and returned to near normal levels by six weeks following the tragic event. An interesting study was conducted by researchers in the New York city vicinity after the September 11 World Trade Center Disaster.[10] Cardiac patients that had implantable defibrillator/pacemakers were evaluated to ascertain the frequency of sensing and firing of the defibrillator. If a patient develops an erratic, deadly heart rhythm, the defibrillator will emit a small electric shock to reset the normal heart rhythm. These devices are part of a pacemaker that is implanted in the chest. Information from the device may be downloaded into a computer to allow doctors to determine the activity of the device. The researchers wanted to examine the activity a few months before and after the disaster. They found that for one month following the tragic event, the defibrillators went off twice as often, but returned to pre-disaster rates by the second month. The researchers postulated that the stress from the daily news triggered the lethal heart rhythms. Without the pacemakers, they would have died.

Other smaller daily frustrations increase stress as well. Anything as simple as a machine that stops working, a flat tire, a missed appointment, a spill on a shirt, a traffic jam, or any number of irritations may trigger stress. How one reacts to the daily frustrations may be an indicator of the level of harm that may be occurring within the body.

Strategies to Cope with Stressors

The first step in battling stressful events in your life is to take care of your body. Exercise, eat right, and get a good night's sleep to be ready for the next day's unexpected events. I described physical activity in chapter 8 and healthy eating tips throughout this book. Getting an adequate amount of sleep is also very important. The American Heart Association recommends that adults should get at least seven hours of sleep every night.[11] If you suffer from chronic sleep interruptions, you should speak with your healthcare provider about it. I've found that a good night's sleep makes almost any problem seem more manageable.

It isn't easy to maintain a quiet calm in the face of a storm, but a positive attitude helps. You may experience a stressful event and rather than deal with it as it happens, you ignore it and bury your feelings and irritations. Each time the problem reoccurs, you continue to ignore it. "After all, it's a small thing. It is better left alone." However, stress is cumulative. You climb a rung on the stress ladder with each negative event that goes unresolved. Once you get to the top of the ladder, the least little thing may throw you over the top and cause you to explode. The adrenalin in your body starts surging. You probably overreact and handle the situation poorly. It would have been better to deal with it in the earlier stages so that your frustrations did not fester and build up to a boiling point.

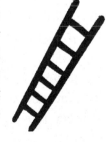

Take a Time Out

At other times, it may be more helpful to walk away from the stressor and take a mental and physical time out. You may find the image of a hurricane helpful. During a storm, dangerous winds swirl around you, but in the very center is an eye of calm and quiet. It doesn't last long, but it gives you a break to gear up for the rest of the storm. When life throws serious stressors at you, take a moment and step out of the storm. You can always escape to the restroom and close the door. No one can reach you there. Just take a few moments to take some deep breaths and clear your thoughts.

Physical Activity

Another strategy for coping with stress is to get moving. This one is especially powerful for me. If I experience one of those moments where my anger is building, it's time to get busy. I clean my house with abandon to help burn off the excess energy and adrenalin. Exercise, a walk, just about anything active will work to distract and calm.

Deep Breathing Technique

Close your door or move to a quiet place. Lean back onto a chair, and if possible, place your feet up. I like to do this exercise by lying on the floor and putting my feet up on a chair or sofa. The blood flows to my brain and increases oxygenation. Close your eyes and take a few deep breaths. Exhale slowly with each one and then inhale slowly and deeply. If you can set a timer and take a short five- or ten-minute power nap, you will be amazed at how refreshed you feel. The adrenalin will begin to leave your body and the stress symptoms begin to abate. Visualize the pounding of the ocean surf or a cool mountain stream.

Relaxation

You can stretch the muscles in your neck by moving your head from side to side slowly. Standing and touching your toes moves oxygen back into your brain. This is really good for fatigue and sluggishness. Go for a brief walk as well. Stretch your arms and legs. It is especially helpful to move in the opposite positions in which you have been engaged. Stand if you have been sitting, etc. Take some deep breaths and try to relax.

Progressive Muscle Relaxation

Sit in a chair or lie on the floor and close your eyes. Begin with your feet and contract your muscles as you inhale and relax them as you exhale. Move up your body with your lower legs, then your upper legs, your buttocks, and abdomen, etc., until you get to your neck. Sit quietly for a few minutes. You should feel more relaxed.

Imagery

Take a five-minute "stay-cation." Close your office door or escape to a quiet place and visualize a beautiful location that you have visited. Think about all of the wonderful, relaxing sights and sounds. It is even more effective if you play the sounds from a CD. Some people find that placing beautiful nature scenes around their office or adding a simple water feature or fountain helps to keep them calm and centered.

Phone a Friend

While gossiping can make many problems worse, it is a good idea to form accountability partners. These are people that you can call who will help you see a situation through their neutral eyes. Often, just verbalizing your frustrations out loud will make them seem much less powerful. Walking with a friend, loved one, or spouse is a great combination of mental therapy, social support, and exercise.

Prayer or Meditation

For me, prayer and reading the Bible help to calm my anxious thoughts more than anything else that I might do. It centers me and helps me to take myself much less seriously. Praying for others is healing. For you, it may be meditation. Whatever your belief, take a few minutes to think outside of yourself and your situation. Another great book that is very helpful is *How to Win Friends and Influence People* by Dale Carnegie. The original book was written in 1936 and updated in 1981. Carnegie teaches you how to look at life through the other person's eyes, which is an invaluable skill for everyone.

Combating Road Rage

For many people, driving stirs up a great deal of stress and anxiety. Exhaust fumes, accidents, construction, and incompetent drivers are just a few of the problems that drivers encounter. The pollution is toxic to your heart.[12] I must admit my frustration levels soar when I'm trapped behind a slow-moving driver in the passing lane. Doesn't he or she realize how much traffic is building up behind them? Move over! A coworker once gave me some great advice for how she dealt with her road rage addiction. First, she stopped playing rock 'n' roll music as she felt that revved her up too much. Next, she changed her mind-set.

> Each time I get in my car, I just assume that every driver I meet will cut me off. I will get stuck behind a dawdler. I expect it. When it happens, I'm not surprised. I tell myself, see, I knew it would happen. I'm just delighted that it hasn't happened more often this day.

As she pulled onto a busy interstate, she was ready. She allowed more time to get to her destinations so that she didn't feel time pressure and the need to swerve in and out of lanes and tailgate. She also changed her music to classical, which soothed her anxious spirit. Her blood pressure improved greatly. Finally, if you encounter an aggressive driver, let them pass. Remember, that they are just a few passing lanes away from a heart attack. Don't let that be you.

Holidays

Sometimes, we think that we have to honor all of the family traditions at the expense of fatigue or illness. Keep your activities simple and enjoy the time with your family and friends. I get the same gift for just about everyone. Finally, if you know that you will be with the liberal Democrat and you are a conservative Republican, pick your battles wisely. A family gathering may not be the best time to have your political debate.

Anger/Hostility

In the 1970s, scientists began to explore how one's personality and manner of responding to life's stressors might impact risk for heart disease. The first to be described was the type A personality by physicians Meyer Friedman and Ray Rosenman in their book *Type A Behavior and Your Heart*. Characteristics are "ambitiousness, aggressiveness, competitiveness, impatience, muscle tenseness, alertness, rapid and empathic vocal style, irritation, cynicism, hostility, and increased potential for anger." (323)[13] It was thought that type A people were at higher risk for heart disease, but early studies were inconclusive. The opposite personality trait was the type B personality described as "even-tempered, patient people who are not at increased risk for heart disease." (265)[14] More recently, a type D or "distressed" personality has been identified."[13] This person may feel inhibited, tense, and insecure around others and avoids social situations. He or she is fearful of disapproval and tends to look at life through a negative lens. Emotions are buried which increases risk for a cardiac event. In short, if you have either a Type D or Type A personality, your health would be improved if you converted to more of an easygoing, positive type B personality.

A scientific review of research conducted between 1983 and 2006 examined the association of anger/hostility with the number of new heart attacks.[15] Approximately, 2,000 people within 25 studies who never had a heart attack and 750 people within 19 studies who had a heart attack were evaluated. While the studies varied, in general, hostility was defined as:

> ...a negative attitude or cognitive trait directed toward others, anger as an emotional state that consists of feelings that vary in intensity from mild irritation or annoyance to intense fury or rage, and aggressiveness as a verbal or physical behavioral pattern manifest in yelling, intimidation, or physical assaults. (936)

The researchers found that angry/hostile men suffered from more heart attacks than their more relaxed, easy going counterparts. Other researchers reviewed 23 studies that taught heart attack survivors better stress related coping skills. Within 2 years following the heart attack, in general, mortality rates decreased by 27 percent and second heart attacks decreased by 43 percent.[16] Learning how to cope with stress was beneficial to their overall health.

Personal Story

Our son played on a Pony League baseball team where my husband served as the assistant coach. The head coach loved the game and volunteered for the league at many levels. While he was a kind man most of the time, he was very competitive and had anger control issues. He overreacted at almost everything and was constantly yelling at his son and the opposing coaches. The worst of his anger was directed at the referees. On more than one occasion, he was ejected from the game. He had a type A (hot-reactor) personality. In contrast, my husband is the polar opposite, slow to anger and easygoing. The only time that you would ever know that he is angry is when he starts to bite his lower lip. He has a type B personality.

One day, the easily angered coach had to leave on a business trip and left the team with my husband. Everyone expected a major defeat since our team had never won a single game and was facing the league's best pitcher on an undefeated team. My husband, ever the optimist, cheered the boys on with positive encouragement for each good play. They caught fly balls, dove for catches, stole bases, hit the ball like never before, and beat the other team 4 to 3. His secret weapon was positive reinforcement. It was a great game and spoke volumes about motivation and the benefits of a type B personality. His coaching style mirrors his life and good health.

Type A coach returned from his trip astonished by the win. However, this story has a tragic ending. His hostile personality killed him because two years later, he died from a massive heart attack at forty-five years old. Everyone was surprised but me. The moral of this story is that if you have a type A personality, know that you are not getting away with it either. Convert to more of a type B personality. Don't sweat the small stuff. When you feel anger and hostility kicking in and your adrenalin surging, don't count to 10…count to 1,000!

A fool gives full vent to his anger, but a
wise man keeps himself under control.
—*The Bible,* Proverbs 29:11

Whether you think you can, or
you think you can't—you're right.

—Automobile Industrialist, Henry Ford

10

Overcoming the Barriers to Change

Y ou are probably reading this book because you are struggling to change a specific behavior. Perhaps a healthcare provider told you to lose weight, quit smoking, or eat healthier because you are at increased risk for a heart attack or stroke. You learned in chapter 1 how a heart attack and stroke develop and the specific risk factors that increase your chance of having an event. You may be concerned and now motivated to make some changes. However, like many people, you have probably tried many times to live healthier, but have become discouraged with failure.

Before you begin, it will be helpful for you to understand the stages that people move through on their way to taking action to change a behavior. Knowing what stage you are in will help you identify strategies that may help you become successful. Experts in helping people change behavior sum up these stages into one word: readiness. What does it mean to have readiness to make a behavior change? Webster's New World Dictionary[1] defines the word "ready" as "prepared to act." From my perspective, readiness involves an entire thought process captured in one question:

"How ready are you to take action to change a behavior such as to quit smoking or lose weight?"

Stages of Change

Psychologists James Prochaska, John Norcross, and Carlo DiClemente[2] did some groundbreaking work in understanding the stages that people move through when altering a given behavior. I would highly recommend their book, *Changing for Good*, if you would like more detailed information on this concept of readiness to change as measured by these stages. The five stages are: Precontemplation, Contemplation, Preparation, Action, and Maintenance (Avoiding Relapse). However, I label them in a simpler manner: Denial, Pros Versus Cons, Taking First Baby Steps, Changing, and Maintaining Change. The stages fall along a continuum beginning from No Behavior Change to Maintaining Change. Relapse could occur at any point and people do not always move in a straight line.

Stages of Behavior Change

No Behavior Change	Maintaining Change
Denial-→Pros Versus Cons-→First Baby Steps-→Changing-→Maintain Change	
* By the author, modified from Prochaska, Norcross and DiClemente, *Changing for Good*	

As you read through this section, think about a single behavior that you are supposed to change and decide which of these stages applies to you. Most people have more than one thing that they need to change. You may find yourself at different stages for various issues. I would recommend focusing on one lifestyle change at a time.

Denial

People in this first stage are generally not interested in changing their behavior. They may not connect the dots between their harmful actions and their risk for a heart attack or stroke. They don't realize that they have a problem. "It won't happen to me." Part of the problem may be that they don't understand how risk factors cause a heart attack or a stroke. The very first step is to truly understand why the harmful behavior is bad, which has been the point of this book. Most people are resistant to give up a harmful behavior that they enjoy, if they don't understand how it is hurting their health.

Suppose your healthcare provider wants you to take a blood pressure medication because she is fearful that you may have a stroke. She tells you "your blood pressure is too high and you need this medication to lower it." You know that high blood pressure is bad, but you feel fine. You don't see any need to take the medication. If you are in the denial stage, it will help you to measure your blood pressures at home. If you record high blood pressure readings, it will be much more difficult for you to remain in denial. The evidence of potential harm may alter your thinking. Your motivation to take the medication prescribed by your healthcare provider will by greater. You have made the connection between the high blood pressure readings and the medication solution to stop the problem.

Personal Story

A few years ago while obtaining my PhD in nursing, I was studying the concepts of "risk taking" and "harmful behavior." We were to go out into the field and observe our concepts in action. I chose to study skydivers. I wore a safety parachute and observed a free fall from the jump plane but did not jump myself. The leader accompanied me up in the plane and told me that most jumpers are in denial regarding potential injuries. If something goes wrong, it was a mistake that the other skydiver made. Most believe that "It won't happen to me because I'm too experienced." His attitude changed when he injured his shoulder the previous week during the free fall and his doctor advised him not to jump again for a few weeks. Despite his resistance, the other members of the team continually cajoled and harassed him to jump with them. It was obvious that he really wanted to jump, but he refused. I thought that it was interesting that the evidence of harm from the pain in his shoulder modified his behavior, even in the face of tremendous peer pressure. This mind-set works to alter attitudes about health-related behaviors as well. People engage in harmful behaviors and may remain in denial until they are confronted with evidence of the "wear and tear" from their actions. Checkups with a healthcare provider who confronts you with that evidence is an opportunity to alter your thinking and enhance your motivation.

If you think that you do "not" need to change your harmful behaviors as suggested by your healthcare provider or you do not understand how your behaviors are harmful, read chapter 1 again. Learning how heart disease develops and the connection with your behaviors may be very helpful for you. Take advantage of screening opportunities described in chapter 2 to determine the wear and tear on your body from your harmful behaviors. The goal is to help you to begin to think about why your behaviors are a problem and how small changes will reduce your individual risk.

Pros versus Cons

People weighing the pros and cons realize that they need to change their behavior, "but" they are very ambivalent about doing it. You may hear them say, "I know that I need to quit smoking, *but* the cravings are too hard to overcome." Or "I know that I need to eat better because my cholesterol is too high, *but* I like food that isn't good for me." People can remain ambivalent, contemplating the pros and cons of changing their behavior for years. Sometimes, physical evidence of damage may serve as the trigger that might push them out of their ambivalence. Discussing the benefits of lifestyle change and overcoming barriers may motivate some people into taking those first important steps.

If you are stuck debating whether or not you should change a harmful behavior, make a list of your pros and cons. "How would your life improve or your heart attack risk be altered if you made this change? Would you feel or look better? What are the costs of making your change? What barriers get in your way?" It may help you to schedule an appointment with a lifestyle coach or consultant who can talk with you about your individual barriers.

Taking First Baby Steps

People who are taking the first baby steps are beginning to change their behavior. They are trying out the new change. A smoker may begin by cutting back on their number of cigarettes, while someone with high blood pressure may chose to stop adding salt to their foods. He or she needs help to ensure that the baby steps are realistic in order to build confidence.

It's very important that the new change be realistic. Let's say that you have set a goal for yourself to quit smoking, lose 50 pounds in 6 months and exercise for 30 minutes every day. All of these goals are laudable but very challenging to accomplish. You may even maintain them for a few days, but most would fail. There are too many changes all at once. A better strategy is to select one thing. Start with a change that you are fairly confident that you can make. How confident are you to stick with your change? Rate your confidence on a 1–10 scale from 1 ("I can't stick with it") to 10 ("I will do it"). Where are you?

Rollnick Confidence Ruler[3]

1	2	3	4	5	6	7	8	9	10

Minimal Confidence   High Confidence

*By author, modified from Rollnick, Mason and Norcross, *Health Behavior Change: A Guide for Practitioners,* 2008

If you say that you are less than 5, you may be trying to do too much. Simplify your plan so that you will be successful. Go slower. Keep it simple and realistic in order to build confidence. Instead of overhauling your diet, begin by adding a fruit and vegetable to it. Instead of joining a gym and exercising every day for thirty minutes, begin with a short ten-minute walk from your house. Some people can dive in and become successful with large changes, but for most people, it is better to go slow and make small changes in your daily life one step at a time. Remember that the most successful lifestyle changes are the ones that you don't notice you are making. They fit more easily into your everyday life.

Changing

The person in this phase is changing his or her behavior. Persons are highly motivated and now ready for the specifics of how to succeed with their new lifestyle. Examples include an eagerness to embrace and learn about healthier eating, joining a gym, or completely quitting smoking. Keep it up! If you are in this stage, congratulations. You are actively changing your behavior! In order to maintain the change, you may need the reinforcement of structured programs to learn how to avoid relapse.

Maintaining Change

True success occurs after six months of making the lifestyle change.[2] Persons are not only changing, but they are maintaining the new change. Success is the gold bonanza! You made it! The new behavior has become a part of your everyday life. However, relapse may still occur. If it is does, be ready for it and then return to the behavior change.

Barriers of Lifestyle Change

Understanding the stages that people move through when changing a behavior is very helpful. However, even with the highest motivation, barriers halt the best of intentions. It will help you to keep moving forward with your behavior change goals by understanding the potential barriers that you may encounter.

Physical Barriers

If you are not feeling well due to an illness, you will be less motivated to change your behavior. Get a good night's sleep as it is easier to face the challenges of the day well rested. Increase your activity, which will raise the "feel good" endorphins in your brain to lift your mood. Eat regular meals to avoid blood sugar drops that trigger cravings, which can sabotage the best of intentions. These behaviors will strengthen your immunity and enhance your wellness. Try some of the following suggestions when you are struggling with cravings.

Stop the Cravings

Wash a car.	Doodle.	Learn a new skill.
Watch a funny movie.	Suck on cinnamon candy.	Go for a walk.
Go to a library or museum.	Eat sunflower seeds.	Wait 15 minutes.
Fly a kite.	Watch a good movie.	Get a makeover or facial.
Get a massage.	Call a friend.	Stretch.
Say a prayer or meditate.	Do your nails.	Do a good deed.
Volunteer somewhere.	Share your feelings.	Renew an old friendship.
Eat an orange slowly.	Sing a song.	Drink some warm tea.
Listen to the birds.	Dance.	Message your temples.
Take a nap.	Deep breathe.	Look at the big picture.
Shop wood.	Wash your car.	Work in the yard.

Lack of Social Support Barrier

Social support refers to having people around you that care about you and support your behavior change goals and has been shown to positively influence behavior change.[4] It involves people who might provide you with tangible assistance, financial support, information, and emotional support. It is also the perception that support would be available if needed. If your family lives a great distance from you, just knowing that they would be helpful in a time of need also counts as social support. The more social support that you have, whether it be in quality or quantity, greatly improves behavior change outcomes.

Social support also involves those who hold you accountable for healthier actions. For instance, a wife concerned about the health of her husband after a heart attack may exert pressure to encourage him to stop smoking. Spousal social pressure has been shown in several studies to improve health outcomes.[4] If you are trying to change a behavior, garner the support of others by telling them about what you are trying to do. Hopefully, when you are having a bad day, they will help you stay on track and encourage you to keep moving forward.

Boredom Barrier

One of the biggest pitfalls for success is boredom. It is a negative mood state, which increases harmful behaviors.[5] Refer to chapter 6 for additional information on this topic. Fill your time with things to do. It will help you keep your mind off of the challenge of exchanging a harmful behavior for a healthier one. Keep your hands, mind, and body busy. You can join a sport's team or club, pick up a needlepoint project. Paint, read a good book, or keep a jigsaw puzzle out to fill your time. Get a part-time job in an area that you love or volunteer. Clean a closet or drawer, work on your car, paint your house, refinish your furniture, or any number of creative ideas to fill your time with rewarding activities. You will be much more successful with your behavior change if you do.

Personal Story

My gynecologist, Dr. James Jenks told me an interesting story a few years ago.

> I see women aging each year as they come in for their annual physical. The ones who see retirement as a time to stop doing all work age very quickly while the ones who find fulfilling things to do age much more slowly. I had one woman who was 99 years old and hoped to work until she was 100. She volunteered as a cook for Meals On Wheels. The last time that I saw her she was upset that we were running behind as she was so excited to get back to her job. An amazing woman!

Keeping busy and active in life has not only kept her healthier, but he noted her wonderful vibrant attitude about life.

Depression Barrier

Depressed individuals tend to withdraw from activities that would improve their lifestyle and was previously discussed in chapter 6. It is important that you speak with your healthcare provider if you think that you may be suffering from depression in order to improve your ability to change your behavior.

Personal Story

I wanted to make the point of the power of depression with an example. I think that many people minimize their chronic sadness when it needs to be addressed. A few years ago, I was working as a hospital nurse on a cardiac floor. It was a Sunday and I was completing tasks following a very busy weekend. One patient with a history of heart problems was hospitalized with chest pain. It was my job to get him ready for his open-heart surgery the next day. He seemed sad and depressed. I don't recall seeing any visitors either. He told me that he didn't think he would make it through his surgery the following day. It was rare for a pre-op patient to verbalize that type of comment to me. I notified the doctor on call for his surgeon and relayed what the patient told me.

I was off for a few days, and when I returned to work, I learned that the patient died during the operation. I saw his surgeon that shift and told him about my conversation with his patient. He was surprised that his partner hadn't notified him of this encounter. The surgeon explained that when a patient verbalizes such a comment, he postpones the surgery. He said he couldn't explain it, but it has to do with the power of the mind and carries a higher risk of complications.

Recently, three patients described different approaches to dealing with their depression. One male told me that the medications caused harmful side effects and he felt that they did not help. A woman told me that the medications helped her tremendously. Another male did not take the medication but filled his life with rewarding activities, which lifted his mood. It makes the point that what works for one person may not work for another. If you are feeling sad or depressed, call your healthcare provider and get evaluated. It will help to increase your behavioral change success.

Poor Quality of Life Barrier

Quality of life is defined as "a person's well-being that stems from satisfaction or dissatisfaction with the areas of life that are important to him or her."[6] If the quality of your life is poor, you will be less likely to engage in healthier behaviors. I studied nearly 200 high risk adults who had three or more major risk factors for a heart attack.[7] The participants were excluded if they already had a heart attack or stroke. I gathered surveys before they were given their results of plaque build-up via a coronary artery calcium heart scan and repeated the surveys three months later. I wanted to explore if the information changed their thoughts and behaviors. The variables measured were: risk perception, health-promoting behaviors, their perception of the benefits and barriers of behavior change, willingness to take prescribed medications, and quality of life. Interestingly, the two variables that impacted the decision to engage in healthier behaviors the most were their "perceived barriers" and "quality of life." As "perceived barriers" increased, health-promoting behaviors decreased. As "quality of life" increased, health-promoting behaviors also increased. My research supported that in order to increase the odds for success at changing a behavior, patients need help to reduce their barriers and improve their quality of life.

Financial Barriers

Some experts have argued that the reason why people do not eat more fruits and vegetables is because they can't afford them. Purchasing cheaper fast food may be more attractive than the more costly lean meats, fruits, and vegetables. Others may avoid physical activity because they can't afford an expensive gym. While cost certainly plays a role, I think that view oversimplifies the complex problem. It ignores other options that are available to help people live healthier lives. A visit to my local McDonalds's revealed that a quarter pounder with cheese meal (large fries and drink) cost $6.19, while a grilled chicken garden salad with a container of milk cost $7.19. Since the healthier choice costs about the same as the unhealthier one, taste may be a more powerful deterrent than cost. Exercise can occur within one's home or a walk around the neighborhood. As one example, a Jazzercise DVD costs $17.[8] Each DVD contains several different workout routines that can be done at home. It may be challenging to live a healthier life while on a budget, but it can be done. A walk outdoors in a safe neighborhood is always beneficial and free.

On the other hand, financial incentives may boost healthier behaviors. Researchers from the Mayo Clinic studied 100 obese employees with BMIs between 30 and 39.9.[9] All groups were exposed to a weight loss educational program. They were randomized into one of four groups: 2 groups that did not receive any financial incentive, 1 group that had to pay $20 if they did not lose 4 pounds in one month, and 1 group was paid $20 if they lost 4 pounds in one month. After one year, 62 percent of the participants who were paid $20 for a 4-pound weight loss per month remained in the program losing on average 9 pounds. Only 26 percent of those who did not have an opportunity to receive the financial benefit lost weight with an average of 2.3 pounds.

The University of Pennsylvania enrolled 878 employees.[10] The participants were given $100 for attending a smoking cessation educational session, $250 for quitting smoking, and $400 if they quit smoking after 6 months and it was validated biochemically. Recall in chapter 7 that cotinine is a marker for nicotine and can be detected within saliva or urine. After 9 to 12 months, 14.7 percent of the participants who were given $400 had quit smoking, while only 5 percent in the information only group had quit. At 15 to 18 months follow up, 9.4 percent who were given $400 remained quitters. Those numbers may seem low, but the annual quit rate is estimated between 4 percent and 7 percent.[11] The researchers calculated that the benefit to employers of having people quit smoking results in an annual savings of $3,400 per employee per year.[10]

Media Barriers

The media also creates barriers. Advertisements alter our cognitive choices both consciously and unconsciously. For instance, consumers know that fast foods are high in saturated fat and salt, which is harmful and will increase cholesterol blood levels and blood pressure. Hesitations to eat unhealthy food are overcome because of the warm family-friendly environment of many fast-food restaurants, lower cost and the taste of the food. In chapter 6, I described the work of psychologist Brian Wansink and mindless eating. Set yourself up for success and be more aware of how unconscious choices impact behaviors.

Environmental Barriers

The environment in which an individual lives and works also influences behavior change. For instance, smoking bans have made tobacco use less accessible, which facilitates cessation.[12] Communities also encourage behavior change through supportive environments. If citizens desire to increase physical activity, safe neighborhoods and parks must be developed. Set up your environment for success. It makes a big difference if you don't have easy access to cigarettes or junk food when you have a craving.

Provider Barriers

Healthcare providers mean well but are not trained to provide lifestyle counseling to their patients. In my doctoral research, I found that most healthcare providers recommend lifestyle changes that are too unrealistic for patients to follow and the patients often fail. The purpose for writing this book was to provide new information about what actually works so that you will be more successful meeting your goals.

In the battle to reduce heart disease, multiple organizations and guideline writers have described the importance of medication adherence, especially in regards to high blood pressure, abnormal cholesterol levels, and diabetes. However, providers may unknowingly create barriers for medication adherence by prescribing medication regimens that are too difficult to follow and include too many side effects. Cognitive impairments or illiteracy among patients also create barriers to following the medication recommendations from the provider. Whether one has a PhD in engineering or a high school diploma, understanding complex medical jargon is difficult. I think that many healthcare providers make assumptions about their patients' medical knowledge that is inaccurate.

The other barrier between the patient and the healthcare provider lies within the quality of their relationship. Some patients are fearful of wasting their physician's time and are too embarrassed to admit their unhealthy behaviors or ask what they perceive are ignorant questions. Many patients perceive that the healthcare provider is not listening to them, even when they do ask questions. In chapter 11, I describe how you can have a stronger working relationship with your healthcare provider. It is important because if lifestyle changes do not control your risk factors, medications may be required. Health outcomes are best when you and your healthcare provider work as a team.

Medication Adherence Barriers

Psychological Barriers

In my experience in working with patients, I have found resistance to taking medication. Far too many people seem to view it as a failure or weakness in their character if they take a medication. One senior citizen that I know epitomized this problem. If she is given one pill that contains two medications rather than the same medications in two different pills, she will feel less reluctant to take it. She views the number of medications a person takes as a weakness. To reduce this psychological barrier, "Polypills" are being considered. For heart attack and stroke prevention, it has been proposed that the single pill would contain aspirin, a blood pressure, and statin medication.[13] The polypill is not a panacea, but it may help improve adherence and reduce risk factors. The reality is that we have no control over the genetic vulnerabilities that we may have inherited. Perhaps a polypill medication will reduce this psychological barrier.

Cognitive Barriers

People are living longer in part because of early detection of medical problems, advanced treatment options, and medications. Cognitive impairment has become a larger problem. Older patients are confused about how to take their medications, the purpose for each one, side effects, and any number of issues. Alzheimer's disease and vascular dementia are conditions that impair memory. If you are the loved one of a patient that is cognitively impaired, be sure that someone goes with him or her for all health-related appointments. It is too easy to misunderstand the healthcare provider's directions. Using a daily pill container will help increase medication adherence, but a caregiver may be needed to dispense the medications accurately.

Illiteracy/Knowledge Deficits Barriers

Illiteracy is defined as "The total inability of adults to read, write, or comprehend information (542)."[14] I've found that medical illiteracy is a more common problem when it comes to misunderstanding healthcare information or jargon. Patients may nod their head that they understand the information when in reality they don't. Ask questions and make sure you understand what your healthcare provider is telling you. Most patients have similar questions when it comes to health-related information. The only dumb question is the one that you do not ask.

Side Effect Barriers

Side effects are a huge barrier for medication adherence. For some patients, it may take several changes to get the right medication and dose with the fewest side effects. Patients may not understand this fact and get frustrated with any drug-related problem that may arise. Abruptly discontinuing medication can cause serous health issues. Contact your healthcare provider before stopping any medication and work together as a team to solve the problem. There are many options available if the first one may not be the best fit or solution.

Cost Barriers

I talked about strategies to reduce medication costs in chapter 3. Don't let this barrier preclude you from taking your medications. Far too often, patients do not pick up their prescription once they discover the cost. Rather than call their healthcare provider for a cheaper alternative, they do nothing. Talk with your healthcare provider, pharmacist, or the manufacturer about your concerns for solutions that will work for you. Most pharmaceutical companies have programs for people who need financial assistance. Speak with your healthcare provider or pharmacist about applying for them.

Complexity of Treatment Barriers

If the treatment plan is too complex, patients will be unable to adhere to it. Taking one pill a day is much easier to remember than a pill that must be taken twice a day. Work with your healthcare provider regarding a plan that works for you. The following strategies may help you as well.

Tips for Taking Medications

Read medication bottles carefully.
Take medications with daily routines: your morning coffee, after brushing your teeth, etc.
Place medications in a visible place such as near your coffee pot.
Place a reminder note on your mirror or somewhere around the house.
Use a daily pill box.
Store medications within a cool dry place, not in the bathroom.
Ask your pharmacist for an easily opened bottle.
Ask your pharmacist for large printed medication bottle labels.
Ask your pharmacist for color coded caps to differentiate your medications.
Place a reminder note on the calendar to remind you of ordering refills 1 or 2 weeks before they run out.
Pack enough medications for your trip to cover any delays.
Read the inserts provided by your pharmacist and understand the purpose for your medications.
Report any side effects immediately.
Maintain follow up appointments to ensure that your medications are working properly.

Take Away Points

Changing behavior is a very complex process with the potential for many barriers to block the very best of intentions. Don't let obstacles alter your plan or goals. If you fall off your path, get back up and try again. It may take several attempts and strategies to get it done. A lifestyle coach can help you work through your challenges and roadblocks. Don't be afraid to reach out to one. As you learned from the stages of behavior change information, begin with small changes to build your confidence. Nothing replaces hard work and persistence to get it done.

Try a new thing you haven't done 3 times.
Once, to get over the fear of doing it.
Twice, to learn how to do it. And a third time
to figure out whether you like it or not.

—Virgil Thomson, American Composer

The art of medicine consists in amusing the
patient while nature cures the disease.

—Eighteenth Century French Philosopher, Voltaire

11

Working with Your Healthcare Provider

Your healthcare provider is a vital member of your wellness team and guides you through the murky waters of medicine. However, all final decisions ultimately reside with you. The ideal relationship between a healthcare provider and patient involves an exchange of information that is easily understood, endorsed, and implemented. It is vital that you understand how to work effectively together as a team. Your family and loved ones serve as the supportive players or cheerleaders on your team. In this chapter, I describe the various members that could make up your health care team and strategies that work most effectively with them to promote health.

Healthcare Providers

When you visit your healthcare provider, you may encounter numerous people who have confusing titles, unclear backgrounds, and uncertain experience. You may wonder, "Is the person taking my blood pressure a medical assistant or a nurse? What is the difference between a physician, a nurse practitioner, or a physician assistant?" The players on the healthcare team seem to be in constant change, which leads to even greater confusion. It is helpful to know that all of the various members of your healthcare team have completed some level of classroom and clinical work. Prior to receiving a license or certification, each healthcare member must pass a national exam. Each state determines their "scope of practice" or exactly the type of care that he or she may provide. The following is a brief explanation of the various team members that you may encounter.

Certified Medical Assistant

When you enter a patient care room, the first person that you encounter may be a certified medical assistant (CMA). He or she may take your vital signs, gather information from you, or perform other basic tasks to prepare you for the appointment. A CMA works very closely with the healthcare provider within the office setting. A high school diploma is required to enter a program, which may take up to one year to complete.[1] Courses of study include basic patient care, communication, pharmacology, nutrition, first aid, laboratory procedures, electrocardiography (EKG) administration techniques, and medical ethics. Upon completion of the program, the candidate must pass a national exam in order to receive certification as a medical assistant.

Licensed Practical Nurse

Some states utilize licensed practical nurses (LPN) more so than other states. An LPN works in a variety of settings, which may include patient homes. In 2010, 29 percent worked in nursing homes, 15 percent in hospitals, and only 12 percent in physicians' offices.[2] The LPN provides the same basic care as the CMA along with some of the tasks provided by a registered nurse. Within an office setting, the LPN works closely with the healthcare provider. Within a clinical setting, the LPN administers all types of medications except intravenous ones and works under the directions of the registered nurse. Courses include English, biology, chemistry, anatomy, and physiology and many of the same courses taken by registered nurses but in a much more abbreviated format. The length of the program varies but often lasts twelve months. Upon completion, the candidate must complete a national exam to be considered licensed.

Registered Nurse

You will encounter registered nurses (RN) at varies stages of your healthcare visit. While an RN may escort you in for your office visit, it will more frequently be a CMA. Sometimes, the RN gathers important history and current problem information to prepare you for the visit with your healthcare provider. In 2008, 62 percent of all RN's worked within a hospital setting.[3] The RN administers your medications including the intravenous ones, performs wound dressing changes and provides patient education. The RN's most vital role is to follow the healthcare provider's directives and implement the plan of care. While all team members diligently monitor for any adverse change within your medical condition, the RN is ultimately responsible for reporting any change in your condition to your healthcare provider. The length of nursing programs vary from two to four years. Prerequisites include courses on English, math, biology, microbiology, chemistry, nutrition, psychology, anatomy and physiology. Basic classroom and clinical coursework within the nursing program includes acute and chronic medical/surgical problems, obstetrics, gynecology, pediatrics, psychiatry, and medical ethics. Students who complete the four-year bachelor of science in nursing (BSN) program take research and additional leadership coursework. The BSN program provides a deeper understanding of the challenges and best approaches in delivering holistic health care not only for the patient but also the family. Many hospitals now require BSN.

Nurse Practitioner

A nurse practitioner (NP) or advanced nurse practitioner (ANP) is a registered nurse who has completed a masters or doctoral level degree. Nurse practitioners learn a holistic nursing perspective that consider the medical as well as social and psychological factors that influence patient behavior and outcomes. By 2015, the NP program will require a doctorate of nursing as the terminal degree.[4] This change has caused a great deal of confusion for nurses, physicians, and the public. From my perspective, this move followed what was happening with other medical professionals such as pharmacists and dietitians that also require a doctorate for the final degree. The changing demands of the nation's complex health care environment require nurse leaders to have the highest level of scientific knowledge and practice expertise. It differs from a medical doctorate. The Doctor of Nursing Practice (DNP) program provides additional knowledge and skills that fosters innovative leadership to enhance the health and well-being of patients and communities. Nurse practitioners are found throughout the healthcare system and may specialize in Neonatal Care (tiny babies), Acute Hospital Care, Primary Care, Nurse Midwife/Women's Health Care, Pediatrics, Adult or Adult Gerontology (elderly) Care. Within the clinic setting, the NP serves as a healthcare provider. If you have a medical problem that requires long-term management, the nurse practitioner may alternate clinical visits with the physician.

Before applying to a NP program, nurses are expected to have clinical expertise and most have experience in intensive care.

It takes four years to obtain the BSN in nursing and another three to four years to complete the NP program. Courses include diagnoses and treatment of conditions within fields of advanced pharmacology, patient health assessment, medical and surgical solutions, pediatrics, psychiatry, obstetrics, and gynecology. Once coursework and clinical rotations are completed the NP must pass a national exam for certification. Each state has different levels of practice guidelines. The NP is licensed by the state and can obtain the ability to prescribe medications. The NP works independently but in some states must have a physician available for collaboration and referral when a problem arises that is out of the scope of the NP's practice.

Physician Assistant

A physician's assistant (PA) functions in a similar manner as the nurse practitioner within the clinic setting. However, their training and philosophy differ when it comes to patient care and community issues. The PA is educated in the medical model system, which focuses heavily on diagnosis and treatment. An undergraduate degree is required to enter a program and may come from a variety of fields while an NP must have a BSN in nursing and clinical experience.

The PA coursework is generally completed in two years followed by one year of clinical work. The coursework is similar to medical school containing classes and rotations in internal medicine, family medicine, pediatrics, surgery, emergency medicine, psychiatry, obstetrics, and gynecology.[5] As with the NP programs, once the coursework and clinical rotations are completed the PA must pass a national certification test. The PA works under the leadership and guidance of the physician and may write prescriptions.

Physician

A physician has extensive education and training in the diagnosis of medical conditions and treatment designed to restore health. In most cases, all of the other members of the medical team work underneath a physician's leadership. When you visit a medical facility, you may only see the NP or PA, but somewhere within the system is a physician for unusual questions regarding your care.

The doctor's education begins with a four-year undergraduate degree. The applicant to medical school must maintain an extremely high GPA and some type of health care experience to be competitive. Medical school takes four years of classroom and clinical rotations covering areas of family practice, internal medicine, obstetrics, gynecology, pediatrics, psychiatry, surgery, and research.[6] Upon graduation, the new physician enters a residency program, which entails an additional four or five years depending on the area of practice. A physician may complete an additional year of practice called a fellowship. National exams are required throughout the process. In order to become Board Certified, the physician must practice a few years within the specialty and pass a written and oral exam.

Communication Tips for a Successful Visit

At any given visit, you could encounter any of these healthcare practitioners. There are a few things that you can do to increase the success of your visit. In chapter 10, I described many of the barriers that impede the relationship between patient and healthcare provider such as embarrassment to ask a stupid question, fear of wasting someone's time, or lack of rapport.

However, you have the most important role to play. If the healthcare provider speaks too fast or uses medical jargon that you don't understand, you must stop and ask your provider to clarify the information. I recommend that you write down your questions in advance prior to your visit. Personally, I find this tip is extremely helpful. I listen so intently that before I know it, I easily forget something that I wanted to speak with my healthcare provider about. But if I have it written down, I can refer to my notes before I leave the office. Do some homework before your visit regarding your situation. In chapter 12, I describe how you can find information on the web that you can trust. Your knowledge and questions will give you a starting point for a discussion of your concerns with your healthcare provider.

Another important factor in your relationship with your healthcare provider is to find a good one. I like medical people that are nice, smart, thorough, and conscientious. I am really fussy about who takes care of me or my family. You are probably thinking, how do you go about finding a good one? I think the best referrals come from nurses or other health professionals who work within clinical settings. Seek them out within your community. As an example, a hospital staff nurse is able to observe how the physician, nurse practitioner, or physician assistant interacts with the other nurses, patients, and family members. The nurse can tell a lot by the type of thoughtful orders written for patient care. Was the healthcare provider rude or cranky when the nurse had to call him or her for an emergency in the middle of the night? Does the healthcare provider follow up with conscientious care if a patient takes a slight turn for the worse? Try to use the healthcare providers that other clinical staff use. Recently, I found an excellent orthopedic surgeon through the recommendation of a physical therapist at a community function. Do your homework and find someone that makes you feel valued and comfortable. Don't let the healthcare providers intimidate you. They are working for you.

Personal Story

My mother-in-law was very ill a few years ago and almost died. She lived in a small river town in Illinois. For six months, she suffered from a horrible rash all over her body. She saw many doctors who could not cure the problem. One specialist was extremely condescending and rude. We took her to the Mayo Clinic in Rochester, Minnesota, and they resolved the problem very quickly. In one day, she saw three specialists. All three were professional, conscientious, thoughtful, and kind. It took some creative medications to cure her problem. The point of the story is do not settle for poor care. Remain diligent. Keep searching for answers until you get resolution. Some medical centers specialize in diagnosing unusual problems. It may take time, but be particular about your healthcare provider. Trust your instincts. If the relationship doesn't feel right, get a second opinion.

Screenings

Another strategy for having a good relationship with your healthcare provider is to maintain regular checkups, screenings, and immunizations. It is much easier to treat problems that are found earlier than later when the problems are much more severe.

The Importance of Dental Hygiene and Flu Shots

You may also be surprised to learn that new research indicates a possible relationship between infections and heart disease. Two areas of investigation have been dental infections and influenza. The importance of dental hygiene, obtaining regular dental checkups, and an annual influenza (flu) vaccination may be more important than previously thought. Again, it is easier for your healthcare provider to treat problems early before they cause untoward outcomes.

Dental Hygiene

Decay of the teeth and gums lead to chronic infections that may worsen underlying plaque build-up within the coronary arteries.[7] The hypothesis is that the harmful bacteria in the mouth are released into the bloodstream triggering the body's defense to eliminate the pathogen. It is well-known that the oral bacteria travel through the heart and damage the heart valves. People vulnerable to this complication are given an antibiotic prior to dental procedures to prevent valve damage. What is unknown is whether the same bacteria worsen the plaque buildup within the arteries of the heart.

A joint statement from the editors of the Journal of the American College of Cardiology and the Journal of Periodontology stated that enough research has emerged that healthcare providers should encourage patients to take better care of their teeth and gums.[8] Periodontists and dentists who see patients with a great deal of oral disease should encourage their patients to follow up with their healthcare provider to determine any evidence of heart disease. While the evidence is still emerging and not completely understood whether or not a true relationship exists, it seems like good advice for all of us anyway. Maintain regular dental exams as described within the guidelines and take care of your gums and teeth.

My dentist has been in the same practice for thirty-four years, caring for patients from childhood through adulthood and end of life. I asked him about a connection between heart disease and poor dental hygiene. Michael Trantow believes that dentists observe the evidence of serious medical problems in the mouth:

> Although the link between poor oral health and the heart is still being studied, I believe there is a link. The heart's blood supply nourishes the teeth and gums. Failing hearts do not pump well. Local mouth infections worsen because of the diminished blood supply and germs flourish easily.

Patients that reach the end of life from aging, cancer or heart problems seem to have a high frequency of "crashing mouth." Despite our best efforts, the gums and teeth can rapidly fail. Do everything possible to keep your mouth healthy. Brush, floss, and see your dentist. You may be protecting your heart.

Influenza (Flu) Vaccination

The same logic may apply to the influenza infection as well. Perhaps there is a connection between the inflammation released from the flu and a worsening of underlying plaque build-up within the coronary arteries, but again, the research is still emerging. No one really knows. However, influenza is deadly, killing thousands of people every year. The infection overwhelms the entire body. Older people or others with compromised immunity have a very difficult time fighting the infection. The American Heart Association and the American College of Cardiology recommend that all patients with any underlying heart disease problem get an annual flu shot.[9] Serious illnesses are very hard on the heart, so keep your immunizations current.

Take Away Points

The prevention of heart disease and stroke begins with a strong working relationship with your healthcare provider. Find one that you can work with and trust. Keep regular checkup appointments, maintain regular screenings and current vaccinations in order to prevent serious disease. Sometimes, when faced with a health threat such as a heart attack or stroke the entire situation may be very frightening and confusing. A health coach or consultant can serve as your patient advocate to guide you through the murky waters of health care. If you need assistance with this service, please visit my Web site at www.living4ahealthyheart.com for more information on our services.

Be true to yourself, help others, make each day your masterpiece, make friendship a fine art, drink deeply from good books especially the *Bible,* build a shelter against a rainy day, give thanks for your blessings and pray for guidance every day.

—College Basketball Coach, John Wooden

12

Research and Web Sites You Can Trust

Just because you hear the words "the study showed" does not mean that you can trust the information that follows. It's hard to imagine a world without the Internet and the plethora of information available at your fingertips. But how do you know which research studies, Web sites, and resources you can trust? In this chapter, I help you understand how to interpret research findings and where to go for good information online.

The Importance of Medical Research

Research is the acquisition of data or knowledge that is obtained objectively. Comparisons are made between the different variables being studied. The Greek philosopher Hippocrates (fourth century BC) was thought to be the first to conduct informal observational studies.[1] He examined how geography, climate, and personal behaviors influenced health in those around him. However, the birth of modern-day medical research probably began with the work of Ignaz Semmelweis, Florence Nightingale, Louis Pasteur, Joseph Lister, and other scientists in the nineteenth century.

Ignaz Semmelweis (1818–1865)

Around 1847, Semmelweis discovered the importance of hand washing to prevent infections in women during childbirth.[2] Pregnant women were admitted to either a birthing suite run by midwives or one run by medical students. Maternal deaths under the care of the midwives was 2 percent, while the medical students had an infection death rate of 18 percent.[2] A close friend of Semmelweis was accidentally cut while conducting an autopsy on a cadaver and died from a similar infection as the women in labor under the care of the medical students. Semmelweis observed that the medical students were going from the cadaver room to the birthing room without washing their hands and were spreading the infection to the women. He instituted a policy of hand washing using chlorinated lime, which decreased the infection rate profoundly from 18 percent to 2 percent.[2]

Florence Nightingale (1820–1910)

Nightingale is known as the Founder of Nursing. She volunteered to care for British soldiers during the Crimean War of 1854 to 1856.[1] She observed the cramped, lice-infested, dirty environments that housed the wounded soldiers. Her meticulous notes and statistics are still admired today. Nightingale cleaned up their environment and death rates decreased from 415 per 1,000 to 11 per 1,000.[1] Nightingale stated, "Put the patient in the best condition for nature to act upon him."(35)[3]

Louis Pasteur (1822–1895)

Napoleon asked chemist Louis Pasteur to solve an alcohol distillery problem in 1863.[4] His scientific examination led to the "Germ Theory." Simply stated, microorganisms cause disease. He heated wine, which killed the microbes, and solved the distillery problem. Today, his pasteurization process is used most commonly in milk. Interestingly, in 1870, the medical community was initially reluctant to embrace Pasteur's "Germ Theory" because it originated from a chemist. However, within a decade, his work on developing a vaccine for anthrax and rabies changed their minds.

Joseph Lister (1827–1912)

Not all physicians were skeptical of Pasture's work. Lister was a Scottish surgeon who noticed that half of his amputee patients died from an infection known as ward fever. He admired Pasteur's discoveries and wondered if microorganisms in the air might be causing the infections. Lister poured an antiseptic onto the wounds of his patients, and within four years, he decreased the mortality rate from 50 percent to 15 percent among the amputee patients.[5] Before Semmelweis, Nightingale, Pasteur, and Lister, surgeons did not wash their hands before surgery nor between patients. Lister experimented on hand washing techniques and the sterilization of instruments. He became known as the Father of Antiseptic Surgery.

John Snow (1813–1858)

An epidemic of cholera broke out in England and persisted from 1813 to 1858.[6] Cholera remains a dangerous and deadly diarrheal disease if left untreated. Snow was a physician who investigated the source of the outbreak. At the time, it was believed that people contracted the disease through the air, which Snow did not accept. He began plotting the individual cases on a map and isolated the source, which was a contaminated water pump. Later, he observed that individuals who lived downstream from the sewage that was dumped into their drinking water had more cases of cholera than those who lived upstream. His work led to changes in sanitation practices and a reduction in the disease.

The work of these early medical researchers changed health care forever. Today, modern-day researchers examine an abundance of medical concerns. Cancer research has exploded with an anti-cancer vaccine around the corner. The human immunodeficiency virus (HIV) responsible for Acquired Immunodeficiency Syndrome (AIDS) was once thought a death sentence, but medical researchers developed medications to control it. Healthcare practitioners base their treatments on the evidence garnered through good research that drives the train of medical progress.

Safe Guards on All Research

To ensure that ethical research is conducted, the Institutional Review Board (IRB) was formed in 1966.[7] Every researcher must get approval from an IRB affiliated with their institution before conducting any research. The IRB consists of a team of knowledgeable, experienced professionals who review the project. Their purpose is to protect the participants from physical or psychological harm. Once IRB approval is obtained, the research subject may be invited to participate within the study. The participant is given information on the purpose of the study, explanation of research procedures, any potential risks and discomforts, benefits, financial issues, what information will be collected, and what will happen to it. Anonymity must be maintained and personal information protected. The participant is reminded that he or she may withdraw from the study at any time. If the individual wishes to participate, a consent form is signed.

If you are invited to participate in a research study, I would highly recommend it. You are part of the process to advance medical knowledge. While the information gathered from the particular study may not help you in the short term, it may help other people in the long run. As with any medical situation, ask a lot of questions and you may find it an interesting experience.

Good Research That You Can Trust

It's interesting to note how many times on the radio or news that you hear "the research showed." The listener is supposed to infer that the study was well done and the results valid. But is it? There are several types of research. However, the most respected and trusted is the Randomized Control Trial.

Randomized Control Trial

The Randomized Control Trial (RCT) is the gold standard for solid research. It contains at least two groups of participants. One group gets the treatment while the other group does not. Both groups are supposed to be similar so that the only difference observed comes from the treatment versus no treatment.

Let's say that a pharmaceutical company has developed a new medication for smoking cessation. The researchers want to test whether the new medication helps smokers quit more so than if the drug wasn't taken. Drug trials go through a very rigorous IRB approval process and generally require a very high number of participants.

Randomization Process

Each participant is "randomly" assigned to one of the two groups and the researcher has no influence or control over the assignment. Randomization may be done any number of ways.

As one example, the researcher puts the same number of red and blue tokens in a hat. The red token is Group A assignment and the blue token is Group B. Each time a new participant is added to the study, either a red or blue token is drawn randomly from the hat and the assignment made. Group A gets the smoking cessation medication while Group B gets a placebo instead. The placebo looks like the smoking cessation medication but only contains sugar. A placebo is used because the process of just taking a pill can alter behavior. If both groups are taking a "pill," this effect will be minimized. Both groups want to quit smoking and attend the same smoking cessation course for six weeks. The only difference is that one group gets the medication and the other gets the placebo. Participants were evaluated six months later for smoking rates.

The Size of the Difference

Once the study is completed, the researcher calculates the average for each group of the number of participants who quit smoking. Statistics are used to compare the difference between the two groups. If there is only a small difference, the study is considered inconclusive. It would mean that the medication had little if any benefit in helping people quit smoking. However, if there were much higher quit rates among Group A who took the medication compared to Group B who used the placebo, the large difference tells the researchers that the medication really did make a difference. Healthcare providers can examine the impact of the study by knowing the statistical number that represents the difference between the two groups.

Sample Size

If researchers found a large difference and it looks like the new medication will help smokers quit, there are a few more things to consider. How many people were studied? Statistically, the results carry more credibility or validity with a larger sample size. The differences observed were more likely due to the smoking medication and not by chance. If the researchers only studied 30 people, then it wasn't a large enough sample to be valid.[7] Drug studies may have thousands of participants while a diet study may have 200 participants. The numbers vary depending on the type of study being conducted. When I look at participant numbers for behavior studies, I want to see larger numbers at least over 100. The point is that very small participant numbers of less than 30 are just not very accurate. An example may help to clarify this point.

Paleo Diet

In chapter 6, I described the Paleo diet. If the hunter/gatherer ancestors didn't eat it, you shouldn't eat it either. Avoid processed foods, etc. Supporters of the diet say that research was conducted and reported in reputable journals that the diet works.[8] The actual studies used a handful of participants with a study duration of a few weeks.[9] While the press release may tout the benefits of this new eating plan, it is hardly enough research to support its effectiveness. The numbers were too small and the studies were conducted for only a few weeks.

Credentials

The final questions to consider involve the credentials of the researchers who conducted the study and the credibility of the author reporting the results. Was there any bias or influence that could impact their findings and reporting? For example, if the person conducting the study gets a financial incentive for prescribing the smoking cessation medication, it could alter objectivity. When reading a research study, it is also important to examine the bias of the journalist reporting the results as well.

Saturated Fat Article

As an example, a controversial article appeared in the *Wall Street Journal* titled, "The Questionable Link between Saturated Fat and Heart Disease" by journalist Nina Teicholz.[10] You might think like others that if it's in the *Wall Street Journal*, it must be true. The author actually stated, based on one review study, "Saturated fat does not cause heart disease—or so concluded a big study published in March in the Journal Annals of Medicine." She went on to say "The fact is, there has never been solid evidence for the idea that these fats cause disease. We only believe this to be the case because nutrition policy has been derailed over the past half century by a mixture of personal ambition, bad science, politics, and bias."[10] You should always be suspicious when one person cites a single study that contradicts a body of research that came to opposite conclusions. The reality is that if you eat a diet high in saturated fats such as butter, cheese, and steak, your LDL (bad) cholesterol should increase along with your risk for a heart attack and stroke.[11] It certainly isn't the only offender but to discount the impact of a high saturated fat diet is not only misleading, it is harmful. Patients may believe that they can eat anything and not worry about the impact on their health. You may view the "American Heart Association Statistical Update: Heart Disease and Stroke Statistics, 2014" for a summary of the most recent nutrition research or visit: http://circ.ahajournals. org/content/early/2013/12/18/01.cir.0000441139.02102.80.

I read the research article that Tiecholz cited, which was a review study. The researchers did a good job collating the information, but the study had several limitations. In a review study, the researchers summarize the findings from a group of studies completed within an area of interest. Statistical analysis is done to see if the group of studies indicated a large difference. In this case, the researchers were looking at a group of diet studies to determine if eating a high saturated fat diet led to heart attacks.

The problem with a review study is that you are trying to compare several different studies together. It's like comparing apples to oranges to grapefruits. They are all fruit but very different types of fruit. Statistical calculations are used to make them a comparison of apples to apples. It's good information for sure but not as accurate as examining a very large randomized control trial like the smoking cessation medication study previously described. I think the findings need to be interpreted with caution and certainly not intended to immediately change practice. More research should be done to see if the conclusions hold up. The authors of the review study actually stated:[12]

> Although the size of the review is in its favor, the limitations suggest that caution is required in interpreting the results, particularly where they conflict with existing research. The authors' conclusions may therefore be too strong, and may not represent the advice given in some cardiovascular guidelines. (3)

The authors of the review study admonished others to use caution when interpreting their findings. However, that is not how the story was reported in the *Wall Street Journal* article.

Hormone Replacement Therapy (HRT) Controversy

Another research-induced problem occurred a few years ago regarding hormone replacement therapy (HRT) in the Women's Health Initiative study. Between 1993 and 1998, nearly 161,800 generally healthy postmenopausal women between 50 to 79 years old from 40 clinical centers throughout the United States were enrolled in the study.[13] Some of the women were randomized to receive a placebo medication or estrogen hormone replacement medication. Progestin was added to the pill in the women who had a uterus. The goal of the study was to ascertain the benefits and risks of taking hormones, a low fat diet, calcium, and Vitamin

D supplements. After five years, the study was stopped because it appeared that the risks outweighed the benefits. The news media reported the danger of HRT based upon the study results. Many patients panicked, physicians discontinued the hormones, and hot flashing symptoms returned with a vengeance. However, a closer examination of the actual numbers provides a more accurate picture of potential risk:[13]

> Over 1 year, 10,000 women taking estrogen plus progestin compared with placebo might experience 7 more cardiac heart disease events, 8 more strokes, 8 more pulmonary embolus (lung blood clots) 8 more invasive breast cancers, 6 fewer colorectal cancers, and 5 fewer hip fractures. (331)

The first thing to note are the small numbers. As an example, there were 7 additional heart attacks out of 10,000 women. Even though this study was well done with a large sample size, 50 percent of the sample were current or past smokers[13] and two thirds were between 60 and 79 years old.[14] On average, most women had been postmenopausal without HRT for 8 years before they began the study.[14] Many of the participants may have already had underlying disease from smoking or advanced age and the HRT had nothing to do with the abnormal outcomes observed. Was the mass discontinuation of HRT really warranted? Rather than panic, each woman should ascertain individual risk compared to benefit when making HRT decisions.

Dr. Marina Johnson, pharmacist, endocrinologist, and expert in menopause treatment, states:[14]

> Denying yourself estrogen does not mean your risk of breast cancer is zero. According to 2005 statistics from the *National Institutes of Health*, among 10,000 women who never took HRT, 30 cases of breast cancer would be expected to occur in 5.2 years. If you compare that figure to 10,000 women who did take HRT, the number of cases of breast cancer increases to 38 cases. (129)

The difference between those who did not take HRT and those who did take HRT was 8 cases out of 10,000 women. Dr. Johnson wrote a very helpful book titled *Outliving Your Ovaries: An Endocrinologist Weighs the Risk and Rewards of Treating Menopause with Hormone Replacement Therapy*. Only 20 percent of women take HRT today. She is concerned that far too many women miss the benefits of HRT: improvements in blood vessels, reduced risk for colon cancer, osteoporosis, Alzheimer's disease, and improved quality of life. She writes:[14]

> For myself, I have decided to take hormones for longer than five years. While my risk for breast cancer and ovarian cancer may be slightly increased, I believe the benefits of HRT and the resulting better quality of life outweigh the risks. However, I must reiterate that this is a very personal decision that each woman needs to make with her own physician based on her own unique situation and risk factors. Understanding the absolute numbers and how they interrelate, instead of just hearing sound bites of an "increased risk," enables you to make a more informed decision. (134)

Dr. Johnson prescribes "bioidentical" hormones that are absorbed through the skin rather than an oral pill. She believes she can prescribe a much lower dose, which is safer and results in much fewer side effects. If you are suffering from hot flashes, educate yourself and speak with your healthcare provider about your options.

I hope by now you will start questioning "the study showed" language. How many people were studied? Who conducted the study? What do the experts within the particular field say about the findings? The answers to these three questions tell you a great deal about the validity, findings, and interpretation of the results. Finally, whenever you hear of a new study, write the information down and ask your healthcare provider about it at the next visit.

He or she will most likely be aware of the controversy and will help you decipher the information. Reliable Web sites may provide you with additional information as well.

Searching the Web

The Internet has really changed how people receive information. There is a wealth of data available on just about every imaginable topic. However, some of the information is not trustworthy. In the following section, I describe organizations and their Web sites that you can trust.

American Heart Association

The American Heart Association (AHA) was founded by six cardiologists in 1924.[15] Their mission statement is, "Building healthier lives, free of cardiovascular disease and stroke. Our mission drives everything we do." The Web site is www.americanheart.org. The Web site is easy to use and full of very helpful patient information.

National, Heart, Lung, and Blood Institute

The National Heart, Lung, and Blood Institute (NHLBI) was founded in 1948.[16] The mission statement is:[17]

> The National Heart, Lung and Blood Institute (NHLBI) provides global leadership for a research, training, and education program to promote the prevention and treatment of heart, lung, and blood diseases and enhance the health of all individuals so that they can live longer and more fulfilling lives.

The Web site is www.nhlbi.gov. There is a great deal of information available. You can view the national guidelines on various topics. Materials in other languages are available as well.

National Guidelines

I wanted to explain how healthcare providers keep up with the changes in research and adjust their practice to reflect the new information. Roughly every ten years or so, experts gather to examine the state of science on a particular topic. They study the most recent, valid research and summarize the new findings. Only the most rigorous research is examined. If the new research inspires them to adjust their practice, they update the guidelines to reflect the change based upon the evidence.

In 2013, a committee reported new research on cholesterol treatment. The members were experts from prestigious medical institutions around the country who primarily treated abnormal cholesterol. They must collectively agree on a particular change in practice before it is placed within the national guidelines. The decisions are based on the research that they review. This practice is common throughout other specialties that meet to review research and form guidelines as well.

On controversial topics, it may be more difficult for the committee to form consensus and issue a joint statement. For instance, a new test may become available and appear to be highly accurate and helpful. It will take time for the research to be completed to test the effectiveness and safety of the new test and then be evaluated by the committee who deliberately, cautiously interpret the evidence. Generally, one study is not enough to change practice. Medicine may appear to move slowly, but it is designed to protect patients. Ultimately, the individual healthcare practitioner must interpret the guidelines as appropriate for each individual patient and situation. You should view the guidelines in your area of concern in a similar manner. They are intended to guide you on a path that the research indicates produces healthier outcomes. Your healthcare provider may discuss with you the reasons for adhering to or altering the guidelines for your individual treatment plan.

Take Away Points

The country doctor of the nineteenth century learned his craft from books and other physicians. Today, medicine and nursing rely on research to determine which therapeutic strategies are most effective. What does the "evidence" or research show? The Web site resources provided within this chapter are based on solid research. The next time that you hear a journalist say, "The study showed," you will know to question it. A healthy skepticism is the beginning of wisdom. Be patient. There is still so much that is unknown and yet to be uncovered.

Other Helpful Web Sites

Centers for Disease Control   http://www.cdc.gov/
National Sleep Foundation   http://sleepfoundation.org/
Portion Distortion   http://www.nhlbi.nih.gov/health/educational/
    wecan/eat-right/portion-distortion.htm
Healthy People 2020   http://www.healthypeople.gov/2020/
    default.aspx

We walk upon Mother Earth from the day we are
born until the day we die. Though many may join
us on our journey, no one walks the same path.

—Agaidika Shoshone Tribal Woman,
Lemhi River Valley, Salmon, Idaho

13

A Word to Healthcare Providers

As healthcare providers, you are on the frontlines of observing the impact of harmful behaviors on health. Unhealthy behaviors cause half of all deaths within the United States.[1] The five diseases most difficult to manage and exacerbated by harmful behaviors are: coronary artery disease, congestive heart failure, chronic obstructive pulmonary disease, asthma, and diabetes. The question remains, what can be done to help patients modify harmful behaviors and replace them with healthier ones? In this chapter, I describe new evidenced-based approaches that have been found to be most effective. The Shoshone tribal woman's quote has relevance for patient care. Many aspects of behavior change have commonalities among all patients. However, each individual patient has a diverse set of problems, barriers, and needs that will require an individualized approach for successful behavior change.

Challenges from the Patient's Perspective

Medical Illiteracy

Medical illiteracy is a learning deficit among patients that creates barriers to following the treatment and medication recommendations from the provider. I have long argued that healthcare providers assume that patients have a much greater medical knowledge base than is actually the case. Do patients really understand the purpose of the treatment and lifestyle recommendations that are prescribed? Complex medical jargon from well-meaning practitioners and rushed time constraints compound the knowledge deficits. The American Medical Association provides an excellent video that shows how patients misinterpret medical information. It can be viewed via the Web site http://www.youtube.com/watch?v=cGtTZ_vxjyA.

An online survey of 1,315 patients with heart disease was conducted by the American College of Cardiology. Researchers asked about the type of information provided by their healthcare practitioner that would reduce their confusion or medical illiteracy.[2] Results indicated:

- (58%) Information about what to expect over time.
- (57%) The difference between normal versus abnormal regarding their condition.
- (47%) The benefits and risks of treatment.
- (30%) Their responsibilities.
- (20%) Videos that help them understand complex ideas.
- (18%) Condition-focused information.
- (16%) Expert commentary.
- (14%) Medication reminders.
- (13%) Peer to peer support resources.

One patient said that "…It would help if they handed you a pamphlet…these are the symptoms, this is what kind of things you should be expecting, this is how to deal with it, and this is what your body is going through" (39).[2] Complicating the issue is that some patients like a great deal of information while others prefer minimal information.[3]

Cognitive Impairments

Dementia is diagnosed in 24 percent of seniors over seventy-one years old and in 38 percent of seniors over ninety years old.[4] Dementia is "a syndrome of acquired persistent cognitive impairment that affects the content, but not the level, of consciousness" (447). Alzheimer's disease accounts for 70 percent of all cases while vascular problems of the brain cause most of the other 30 percent.[4] Many adults with milder forms of dementia compensate very well and appear to have higher brain function than actually exists. The only way to really tell if the patient comprehends medical advice is with a "return demonstration" or "teach back" technique.

I counseled over 1,000 patients regarding their results following a coronary artery calcium (CAC) heart scan. Recall from chapter 2 that the test measures the quantity of plaque building up within the arteries that surround the heart. I used the "teach back" technique to ensure that the patient understood the findings and the appropriate follow up. One comment that worked well, "Mr. Jones, we talked about many things today. Please tell me how you will describe your results to your friends or family." The response provided a great deal of information about comprehension and retention. If Mr. Jones remained confused, the misconceptions could immediately be corrected before he returned home.

Keep your medical regimens as simple as possible. Avoid medical jargon and use terms that are easily understood. Test comprehension with the "teach back" method. Provide the patient with printed information or write the instructions on paper.

Encourage a family member who is not cognitively impaired to come with the patient for office visits as well.

Personal Story

We noticed that one of our close relatives was becoming more forgetful. She was eighty-two years old at the time and we were concerned about issues related to self-care, medication adherence, and driving. She underwent thorough memory testing at the Mayo Clinic, which involved a magnetic resonance imagery (MRI) test of the brain and a battery of tests to measure her mental and functional capacity. She compensated for her cognitive impairments extremely well and initially fooled the neurologist regarding her level of dementia. However, the MRI indicated a great deal of damage and revealed her deficits. The neurologist told her that she shouldn't drive and would benefit with an assisted living arrangement to help with her care and medical management. He said that her daily crossword puzzle habit had protected her brain and accounted for the compensation that had been observed. The point is that many patients hide their knowledge deficits. The "teach back" technique may help to ascertain the level of cognitive impairment that may be present.

Depression

Depression is present in 4 percent of the general population and 20 percent of those with coronary heart disease.[5] Many others have depressive symptoms and are vulnerable to a worsening of the disease. Recently, the American Heart Association (AHA) released a statement that depression should be considered a serious risk factor that worsens heart disease. When major depression coexists with chronic conditions, morbidity, mortality, visits to the healthcare provider, and emergency room (ER) visits increase, along with days spent in bed and disabilities.[5] In addition, fewer patients participate in cardiac rehabilitation, risk factor modification is reduced, and quality of life impaired. Cardiologist Alan Rozanski studied patients following a cardiac event.[6] He found that patients with negative mood states such as anxiety, stress, pessimism, hostility, or depression were reluctant to engage in healthier behavior change activities following their events. He advocated that clinicians treat negative mood states before initiating lifestyle counseling.

Healthcare providers working with patients who have heart disease should screen for depression using the Patient Health Questionnaire.[5]

Patient Health Questionnaire 2 (PARQ-2)[5]

Over the past 2 weeks, how often have you been bothered by any of the following problems?
1. Little interest or pleasure in doing things. 2. Feeling down, depressed, or hopeless.
If the answer is "Yes" to either question, then refer for more comprehensive clinical evaluation by a professional qualified in the diagnosis and management of depression or screen with PARQ-9.
Patient Health Questionnaire 2 (PARQ-2) *American Heart Association Science Advisory Depression Screening

You may obtain a copy of the longer nine question (PARQ-9) form by visiting the following link: http://www.integration. samhsa.gov/images/res/PHQ%20–%20Questions.pdf.

Asymptomatic Nature of Disease

Conditions such as hypertension, dyslipidemias, and the progression of atherosclerosis occur silently without symptoms. Patients are reluctant to take medications for asymptomatic problems, which leads to a great deal of denial of the danger. Qualitative researchers investigated women's perceptions following a cardiac event via a "phenomenological study."[7] This type of study, examines experiences through the perceptions of the people involved. The insight of the women who were interviewed highlights the problem. Three themes emerged: "Out of sight, out of mind," "Why doesn't he talk to me like that?" and "It's scary."

Out of Sight, Out of Mind

It appeared that once the blocked arteries were opened, the heart problems were gone. The women didn't feel sick and didn't view coronary artery disease as a chronic problem.

> I've done great. I mean I don't consider myself with heart disease. I don't consider myself sick…I mean, I don't feel sick…I think I had something that was fixed, and I'm okay now. Um, I feel better now than I did when I was 35…I'm not going to worry about it. If something comes up…I'll go see about it. (p. 437)

Why Doesn't He Talk to Me Like That?

Women also expressed information regarding the quality of the relationship with the physician.

> I sort of just got ignored. And I think that comes with being a woman…45. And they just more or less ignored me because I think they thought it was just nerves or, you know, something like that. (p. 439)
>
> I heard him talking to a male in the room next door, and he was saying how glad he was to see this guy and how he was looking good, and…I thought, well…he has a relationship with the man…It just made me wonder why he didn't talk to me like that…He just didn't seem to have the same care for me…maybe it's because I'm a woman. (p. 439)

It's Scary

The women were very frightened from the cardiac event. This fear may be so overwhelming that it is easier to ignore any risk of danger for another event rather than deal with the barriers of behavior change.

> Most people don't understand how frightening it is to think that you may not be here next year. Or that you may have a heart attack and ...be an invalid. Because that's something you have to think about. (p. 440)

The asymptomatic nature of atherosclerosis allowed the women to ignore potential risk or danger for another cardiac event. Healthcare providers need to reinforce the importance of controlling risk factors at every visit. More importantly, the women highlighted the importance of building rapport so that patients feel comfortable discussing their fears, knowledge deficits, and barriers.

Challenges from the Healthcare Provider's Perspective

A survey of 547 US cardiologists and 129 care team practitioners was conducted by the American College of Cardiology. Clinicians stated that the three biggest challenges that they face in improving patient health involve weight loss (92%), medication adherence (90%), and exercise (87%).[2] Other issues that are challenging include improving diet, smoking cessation, the complications from other co-morbidities, poor insurance coverage / access to care, and lack of motivation. They also found that patients believe that they are taking better care of themselves than reality suggests. One patient stated it best.[2] "I would give myself a 3 (on a 1–5 scale) and I know my cardiologist would give me a 2. My numbers are good, but every time I go, I just lose enough weight so he won't yell at me." (36)

Clinical Inertia

Healthcare providers may feel frustrated with these challenges, which can lead to "clinical inertia," defined as a failure of the healthcare provider to initiate or intensify therapy when indicated.[8] Clinical inertia is especially problematic when it comes to behavior change. Researchers from one study found that approximately 86 percent of physicians advise their patients to quit smoking, but only 17 percent follow up to monitor progress with quitting.[9] Only 65 percent of primary care physicians advised their moderate/severe obese patients to lose weight.[10] The physicians cited lack of training, time, patient materials, and reimbursement as other reasons for not initiating lifestyle counseling.[10] There may be solid reasons for the healthcare provider to decide to refrain from following national guidelines for patient care. It's important to remember that the guidelines were written as a "guide" for the healthcare provider. The final decision should be left up to the practitioner based on the knowledge of each individual patient. However, knowledge deficits regarding the appropriate approach to complex patient problems may explain some of the hesitation. Insight into behavior change may help to overcome this practitioner barrier.

Stages of Change

Psychologists Prochaska, Norcross, and DiClemente described five stages that patients move through on their way toward behavior change: Precontemplation (Denial), Contemplation (Weighing the Pros Versus the Cons), Preparation (Taking Baby Steps), Action (Changing), and Maintenance (Maintaining Change). I relabeled them to make it easier to follow. The stages of change information is helpful, but it is important to remember that patients do not always move in a straight line. They may be in one stage for one behavior and another stage for something else. Refer to chapter 10 for additional information.

Stages of Behavior Change

No Behavior Change	Maintaining Change
Denial-→Pros Versus Cons-→First Baby Steps-→Changing-→Maintain Change	
* By Author, modified from Prochaska, Norcross and DiClemente, *Changing for Good*	

Precontemplation or Denial

The person in denial may not know that a particular behavior is harmful to health or is aware of the health risk but does not have any interest in changing a harmful behavior. This patient is resistant to changing and often defensive. Rolling with their resistance and gently tying their actions to adverse health consequences may help move them out of this stage. I found that evidence of subclinical atherosclerosis build up from a coronary artery calcium heart scan was very powerful in moving patients out of denial. Patients resisting hypertension medications may find tracking their blood pressures at home helpful. As the patient observes the higher numbers, they may be less resistant to the need for medication.

However, if the healthcare provider pushes for behavior change such as directing the patient to sign up for a smoking cessation class, begin a daily exercise class, or join a weight loss program, the message may be overwhelming and perceived as nagging. These behaviors are of course important things to do, but this is not the time to send that message. It will only lead to more denial and resistance. Gently make a case for the needed change, roll with their resistance, and don't push too hard. Give the patient time to consider the options and the information.

Contemplation or Weighing the Pros versus the Cons

This stage represents a person who is ambivalent about making a change. People can languish in this stage for years. It will help them to make a list of the pros and cons of changing. Benefits versus risks of doing nothing conversations may be very helpful. Be sure that the patient understands the rationale for treatment.

Preparation or Taking Baby Steps

Preparation or Taking Baby Steps refers to the person who is trying out the change. In order to build confidence, people need to start with small realistic changes. A sedentary person may find a gym membership and exercise prescription for thirty minutes on most days of the week overwhelming but a ten-minute walk from the house more realistic. The Confidence Ruler may help the practitioner ascertain if the steps that the patient planned to take are realistic.[3] "How confident are you that you will succeed with your change? Ask yourself on a 1–10 scale from 1 ('I won't succeed') to 10 ('I will do it'). Where are you?"

Confidence Ruler

1	2	3	4	5	6	7	8	9	10

Minimal Confidence   High Confidence

*By author, modified from Rollnick, Mason and Norcross, *Health Behavior Change: A Guide for Practitioners,* 2008

If the patient says that the level is less than 5, the behavior change may be too difficult to do. Help the patient to rethink the plan so that he or she will be successful. It must be kept simple and realistic in order to build confidence. Success with one small change leads to success with other changes.

Action or Changing

This person has a high level of motivation and is making changes in his or her behavior. Information on how to maintain the change will be greatly appreciated. This person will be more interested in a smoking cessation course, actively participating in an exercise program, or interested in joining a Weight Watchers Program to lose weight. This individual is highly motivated to make changes in his or her life.

Maintenance or Maintaining Change

When the person has maintained the new behavior for at least six months, he or she has entered the maintenance stage. Help your patient develop strategies that cope with potential relapse. Refer him or her to support groups, which may be very helpful.

It is interesting to note that of people who need to change a harmful behavior, only 20 percent have enough motivation to actively alter their lifestyle.[11] The other 80 percent are trapped in the other stages: "Denial, Weighing the Pros versus the Cons, or Taking the First Baby Steps." I call these "Non-action" stages. For the healthcare provider, it is important to remember that each stage requires a different approach to enhance motivation. If a well-meaning professional provides information that is too unrealistic or inappropriate, the person mired in one of the non-action stages often becomes angry, defensive, or overwhelmed by the recommendation. This person may nod their head and appear to agree with your recommendation but may leave the office, knowing that they will not be able to adhere to it. The person may even try out the recommendation for a short bit of time but ultimately fail. The recommendation must be based on the individual's stage of readiness to change, be realistic and simple, or the medical advice will not work.

As I examined the research on behavior change, I found that nearly all lifestyle advice was too challenging and unrealistic for most people to follow. One example comes from the latest weight loss guidelines.[12] For weight loss, women should restrict calories to less than 1,200 to 1,500 a day and men less than 1,500 to 1,800 a day. Aerobic exercise should equal thirty to forty minutes on most days of the week. Weight loss research supports these recommendations and the patient would certainly lose weight if followed. For the 20 percent of people who are motivated and are in the "changing" stage, they would be open to implementing this advice; however, everyone else would be overwhelmed. Most overweight people can't make these drastic changes all at once. It's just too much too fast. I argue that this advice is unrealistic and a simpler approach is needed to lead people to weight loss success. This book was written for those individuals within the 80 percent who struggle with changing harmful behaviors. I hope they learned that all changes, including small ones count.

Motivational Interviewing Techniques

Motivational interviewing (MI) is a counseling technique that was developed by psychologists Stephen Rollnick, Pip Mason, and Chris Butler working within the world of addictions counseling. MI can be used during brief encounters with patients and has been shown to enhance smoking cessation rates[13] and physical activity participation.[14] It is a patient-centered collaborative interaction that rolls with the resistance of the individual, gently makes the case for the importance of change and builds self-efficacy to facilitate the change. The healthcare provider uses a "guiding" style rather than a "directing" style to help the patient decide which healthier changes they wish to make. Rollnick, Miller, and Butler wrote:[3]

> It is within this "spirit" of motivational interviewing that the three communication tools come together to guide, rather than badger, to encourage rather than shame, to negotiate rather than dictate. (116)

Building Rapport

The most important component of MI is to build rapport with the patient and begins with the initial patient contact. The following common interaction provides insight into those things that sabotage rapport.[3]

> Next, please [after a 1–hour wait in a full waiting room]. Thank you, Ms. Evans. Can I ask you to please get undressed to your underwear and put this gown on? I'll come back and do your vitals, okay? Then you'll see the nurse and then...? (157)

It isn't clear whether the staff introduced themselves before asking the patient to disrobe. However, the depersonalization is hard to undo and sets the stage for a poor interaction. Some patients are fearful of wasting their physician's time, are too embarrassed to admit their unhealthy behaviors or ask what they perceive are ignorant questions.[15] Many patients perceive that the physician is not listening to them, even when they do ask questions. The simple things really count here. It's important to remember that if the receptionist, medical assistant, nurse, or any other staff member is unkind, it will impact the relationship between the patient and the healthcare provider. Staff should always introduce themselves to the patient and family upon entering the room. Create a situation where the patient feels safe, that the healthcare practitioner genuinely cares about his or her well-being and that good care will be provided. The extra steps help the patient feel more comfortable and strengthen rapport.

Overcoming Ambivalence and Poor Self-Efficacy

When using MI techniques, the healthcare provider gently makes the case for the needed change. Barriers are discussed, and ultimately, the patient determines the type of lifestyle change that will be made. Small steps are encouraged to build self-efficacy. Success with the smaller changes leads to additional changes. If the patient does not have confidence in their new behavior, relapse is common. The Rollnick Ruler is used to determine confidence levels as previously discussed. The following dialogue is a good example of MI:[16]

Example of Motivational Interviewing

Patient	*I wish I didn't eat so much fast food.*
Practitioner	*You eat fast food fairly often.*
Patient	*Pretty much every day. I know I shouldn't, but it's just easier.*
Practitioner	*It's easier because you don't have to plan and cook meals.*
Patient	*And I can just run over to the drive-through.*
Practitioner	*So you don't want to give up the convenience of fast food, but you would like to eat healthier.*
Patient	*Right…I guess there are some healthier items on the menu.*
* Encouraging Patients to Change Unhealthy Behaviors with Motivational Interviewing," *Family Practice Management*	

The practitioner is using open-ended statements and reflecting back what the patient is saying. The tone is empathetic and kind. Finally, the "patient" comes up with a solution to the problem. It may seem like a small change, but the patient is beginning to think differently about eating fast food. A few statements that I find particularly helpful to enhance the conversation:

- Tell me what brings you here today.
- Tell me what you understand about high blood pressure.
- If you had to change one thing, what would it be?
- Can you describe what worked in the past?
- What barriers got in your way of meeting your goal?
- How confident are you that you can make this change on a scale from 1 to 10?
- It sounds like you had trouble making this change.

The open-ended statements stimulate conversation. The patient should be doing most of the talking and eventually comes up with the solution of what they wish to change. Three key points that sum up motivational interviewing are:[3]

- Ask where the person wants to go and build rapport.
- Inform about options and ask what makes sense to them.
- Listen and respect what the person wants to do and offer help as needed.

If you would like to learn about motivational interviewing training you may visit: www.motivationalinterviewing.org or read *Motivational Interviewing for Health Care*. Rollnick, Miller, and Butler wrote:[3]

> In the consultation about behavior change the most important element...is what we called the "spirit" of the conversation, where a guiding style is used to elicit from the patient their own good reasons for change. (175)

Personal Story

For me, the most challenging piece when using the MI techniques is allowing the patient to determine the changes to be made. I had a three-pack-a-day smoker that had a very abnormal coronary artery calcium heart scan. The test detected a great deal of subclinical atherosclerosis (plaque) in several coronary arteries. While he hadn't had a heart attack or stroke yet, he was at very high risk for one. In addition to smoking, he had multiple risk factors as well. In my mind, his smoking was the most dangerous problem and the priority for change.

However, he decided to increase his physical activity and continue to smoke. He articulated that his life was too stressful and he couldn't quit. Astonishingly, a few months later, he called me to say that he had quit smoking. He cited two reasons for his success. First, he couldn't forget the image of the trauma each puff was causing to his arteries as I had described in our meeting. He always knew that smoking was bad, but once he saw the plaque build-up, it all became more of a reality and concern for him. Secondly, he decided to increase his exercise, which helped him manage his stress better, enabling him to finally quit smoking. As I have said throughout this book, it all comes down to what the individual person is willing to change. Our job is to gently guide the patient through the process.

The 5 As

Another approach that helps providers work with patients is to follow the 5 As that were described within the smoking cessation guidelines.[13] They are a simple acronym to remind busy clinicians the key points in helping patients quit smoking, but they may be used with other behaviors as well.

- Assess the need to change behavior.
- Advise the individual to modify their harmful behavior.
- Agree upon treatment and lifestyle goals.
- Assist the patient with behavior change.
- Arrange follow-up to provide support for continued change.

Enhancing Medication Adherence

In the battle to reduce cardiovascular disease, multiple organizations and guideline writers have described the importance of medication adherence, especially in regards to hypertension, dyslipidemias, and diabetes. However, providers may unknowingly create barriers for medication adherence by prescribing regimens that are too difficult for patients to follow and include unsatisfactory side effects.

A study evaluated 6,748 patients from 31 hospitals across the nation who were discharged after having an acute myocardial infarction or heart attack between 2003 and 2008.[17] At discharge, 93 percent were taking a beta-blocker for blood pressure, 88 percent were on a statin for cholesterol reduction, and 88 percent were on an ACE inhibitor or angiotensin-receptor blocker (ARB). These medications are considered standard of care following a heart attack.[18] Unfortunately, after 12 months, only 12 percent of patients were taking the beta-blocker at the appropriate dose, 26 percent for statins, and 32 percent for ACE inhibitors or ARB's.[17] An abundance of research supports the use of these medications to prevent a second heart attack. However, adherence remains a major problem.

Tips to Improve Medication Adherence

Healthcare Provider
Assess cognition and social support for taking medications properly.
Educate the patient and family regarding the importance of the medication.
Reinforce the risks and benefits of no medication versus drug therapy.
Encourage the patient in the decision making process.
Simplify the regime as much as possible.
Utilize drug combinations whenever possible: the fewer the pills the better.
Prescribe a larger dose and have the patient take ½ of the pill to cut costs.
Describe what to do if a dose is missed.
Schedule follow up appointments before the patient leaves the office.
Reinforce Patient Teaching Points
Read the package information provided by the pharmacist.
Take the medication as prescribed.
Use a pillbox with days of the weeks and slots for times in the day.
Place a reminder near the coffee pot or bathroom when to take the medications.
Report any side effects "before" stopping the medication.
Do not store medications in the bathroom.
Allow 2 weeks to refill medications so they do not run out.
Mark the calendar when refills are due.
Take enough medications for trips. Allow for extra days if the return is delayed.
Order easy twist tops for seniors with disabilities.
Order color coded tops for different medications.
Call the pharmaceutical company if you need financial assistance with your medication.

Preventive Cardiovascular Nurses Association

You may find excellent resources for your patients through the Preventive Cardiovascular Nurses Association (PCNA) established in 1992.[19] It is an international organization of nurses and other healthcare professionals that supports evidenced-based cardiovascular practice. The mission statement includes "developing and promoting nurses as leaders in this field and supporting comprehensive risk reduction strategies for individuals and populations across the lifespan."[19] Their Web site is www.pcna.net. You will find a myriad of resources for you and your patients. Cardiovascular leaders from across the nation are invited to speak at the annual convention to provide the latest evidence that impacts cardiovascular care.

Johnson Research Study[20]

I wanted to provide you with information about my doctoral dissertation research since it is related to the topic of behavior change. The study was titled: "Risk Perception, Psychological Well-Being, and Health-Promoting Behaviors in Persons Informed of a Coronary Artery Calcium Score." The purpose of the study was to examine "how the awareness of a CAC score altered risk perceptions, psychological well-being and health-promoting behaviors in persons at high risk for cardiovascular disease (CVD)" (58).

The study used a descriptive, prospective design with 174 high risks adults with three or more major risk factors for CVD. Scientifically validated surveys were used to measure risk perception, quality of life, health-promoting behaviors, the benefits and barriers of behavior change. Participants were asked about their medication use, risk category, and level of worry. In addition, open-ended questions were provided to allow the participants an opportunity to share additional feedback. The surveys were administered "before" the individuals knew their results and three months following their CAC scan.

Participants were divided into five groups based on their CAC score findings: 0 = no risk, 1–10 = low risk, 11–100 = mild risk, 101– 400 = moderate risk, and over 400 = high risk for a stenotic lesion. Of the participants, 74 percent had some amount of calcium deposition in their coronary arteries from very small scores to very high abnormal scores. This finding was not unexpected as subjects had three or more major risk factors for heart disease. Most participants (68 percent) identified their risk category accurately and 76 percent were concerned enough about their results to follow up with their healthcare provider. However, an area of concern was that only 24 percent within the highest risk group (CAC over 400) stated that they were at higher risk.

Quality of life scores were unchanged before and after the scan ($p=0.06$). Worry levels decreased among three groups, normal (0 CAC) risk group ($p=<0.001$), low (1–10 CAC) risk group ($p=0.01$), and mild (11–100 CAC) risk group ($p=0.01$). Critics of the technology have argued that knowledge of subclinical disease would lead to anxiety and worry. However, our study indicated that quality of life remained unchanged and in the lowest three CAC groups, worry levels significantly decreased from baseline to the three-month follow-up. Health-promoting behaviors increased in all five groups ($p<0.001$). Chi square analysis indicated that medication use increased for lipids ($p< 0.001$) and aspirin use ($p< 0.001$). The CAC score information appeared to enhance motivation to take the medications recommended by their healthcare provider. The two strongest predictors of health-promoting behaviors were perceived barriers ($\beta=-0.41$; $p<0.001$) and quality of life ($\beta = 0.44$; $p<0.001$). As perceived barriers increased, health-promoting behaviors decreased, and as quality of life increased, so did health-promoting behaviors.

Responses from the open-ended questions added validity to the quantitative findings.

> I was struck with concern and fear of my predictable future of illness if I didn't do something about my buildup (female, 67 years old, CAC score of 5).

> This is a wake-up call. Time to look into all the risk factors (male, 50 years old, CAC score of 276).

> Accepting that your vulnerable (female, 63 years old, CAC score of 134).

> I was concerned and the scan confirmed it. The scan saved my life (male, 62 years old, CAC score of 2,736)!

Recall that a calcium score is a marker for subclinical atherosclerosis disease.[1] Healthcare providers should follow the guidelines of the American Heart Association and the American College of Cardiology and encourage their patients at intermediate risk or persons with three or more major risk factors to obtain a screening non-contrast scan to identify those at risk for a cardiac event.[21] Clinicians should ensure that patients understand their results. Awareness of an abnormal finding may provide a "teachable moment" to increase motivation to alter harmful behaviors. We found that a picture is worth a thousands words. Patients may be more willing to adhere to medication prescriptions and modify harmful behaviors in order to reduce cardiovascular risk in the presence of subclinical atherosclerotic disease. Practitioners should ask patients about perceived barriers and poor quality of life, which may impede behavior change.

Take Away Points

Lifestyle change is a complex problem for healthcare providers and patients. Changing a harmful behavior and replacing it with a healthier one is much easier said than done. The silent asymptomatic nature of subclinical atherosclerosis, hypertension, dyslipidemias, or diabetes makes it more difficult for patients to accept that they may be at greater risk. However, the response from the healthcare provider can greatly enhance outcomes. The clinician plays a pivotal role in taking advantage of the teachable moments. Learning about new tests that determine risk and techniques that enhance behavior change are vital to help patients. Practitioners may enhance change by building rapport, rolling with patient resistance, making a case for the needed change, and allowing the patient to determine the behavior that will be changed. Working with patients to modify harmful behaviors and replace them with healthier lifestyles will be the great challenge for practitioners in the new millennium.

> He who cures a disease may be the skillfullest, but he that prevents it is the safest physician.
>
> —Seventeenth Century, English Theologian, Historian and Author, Thomas Fuller

The difference between winners and losers is that
winners do things losers don't want to do.

—Psychologist and Television Personality,
Dr. Phillip McGraw

14

Closing Thoughts

In closing, I wanted to share the stories of three people who struggled with overcoming a harmful behavior and conquered it. May each story help you to think differently about your situation and enhance your motivation as you embark on your own journey.

Linda's Smoking Cessation Story

Linda grew up in a home where both parents smoked as did many of her friends. She began smoking at age nineteen in order to fit in and quickly enjoyed the habit. Among her many triggers were the early morning cigarette upon waking, unwinding after work, and fellowship with other smokers. Doctors encouraged her to quit, but she enjoyed the habit too much. She tried the medication Chantix for two years, which she stated, "It made the cigarette taste awful. I just kept changing brands to find one that didn't taste bad so I could keep smoking. Chantix didn't help me quit." While she tried to quit smoking a few other times, it took a painful and frightening event to stop. Linda was hospitalized with what she describes as "walking pneumonia."

> It was the Christmas sickness in July. I was short of breath and had severe pain in my lungs every time I took a breath. It scared me as my mother died from lung cancer and I outlived her by twelve years. I knew that it was time to quit. My daughter told me about an antidepressant medication that might help, so I tried it. Zyban stopped the nagging cravings. They would last for only ten seconds, then go away. I quit smoking three years ago on July 25.

Linda enjoys the money that she is saving by not smoking, the support from her family and friends and mostly the sense of accomplishment from beating a forty-year pack-a-day smoking habit.

Philip's Weight-Loss Story

Philip says that he grew up lean and active. His battle with weight began with a work-related benefit at twenty-nine years old. Initially, his company provided a food allowance of $35 per day while traveling on company business. He could pocket any money that was not spent on food. Philip ate breakfast at the hotel, then ordered simple meals such as a $5 Subway sandwich for lunch and dinner. However, the company increased the food allowance to $50 a day and any money not used for food could not be pocketed. He recalls:

> It was a disincentive. What I didn't spend I couldn't keep. So I ate it up. I ordered an appetizer, dessert, extra beer, or wine. I wanted to spend my $50 benefit. The pounds started adding up. My weight ranged from 172 after a bout with mono to 217. The funny thing was that I didn't see myself as a fat person. My girlfriend, now my wife,

is a nurse practitioner and she was concerned about my health as my blood pressure was rising. I started to make some changes and lost 15 pounds but relapsed and began gaining weight again. It took a great deal of courage for my wife to tell me, "Philip, you are getting fat again." I needed to hear those words and they changed my life.

Philip investigated weight loss programs and began working with a trainer who pushed strenuous exercise and a restrictive diet. He ate grass-fed lean meats and vegetables while avoiding processed foods, dairy products, and whole grains. The change in his exercise and eating worked. He lost the weight, his blood pressure improved, and he stopped snoring. He maintains his weight loss by choosing foods from the cafeteria salad bar at work.

Most people would find Philip's approach too challenging to maintain, but for some people, it does work. I'm also concerned about the nutrients that he may be losing by giving up whole grains and low-fat dairy products. While I do not recommend this aggressive program to my patients, his story is a reminder that everyone will have a different approach to lifestyle change. For most people, simple changes are the more realistic way to begin a weight-loss program.

Judy's Weight-Loss Story

Judy said that as a child, she was a bit overweight and described herself as a "sturdy little child." However, at six years old, the family doctor encouraged her parents to take her to an endocrinologist who placed her on an extremely restrictive 600-calorie diet. She says that she struggled with excess weight much of her adult life. "I walked at least two miles a day, but it wasn't enough to keep the weight off." While in her forties, Judy was diagnosed with rheumatoid arthritis. Faced with a heavy medication regime, Judy decided to change her exercise and eating. Today in her seventies, she participates in an aerobic and resistance class two times per week. She described her exercise class experience.

> I'm the oldest person in the exercise class. It pays off because I feel great and I'm more active than most of my peers my age. However, I do wonder when they are going to put me in "silver sneakers" before they let me exercise.

Judy line dances for five hours each week as well. She eats lean meat with a little bit of protein at every meal and a handful of almonds every day. She avoids processed foods and fills her diet with mostly fruits and vegetables. She also believes that it is imperative to get eight hours of sleep every night. Judy summarized her motivation to maintain such an active lifestyle:

> We will all die one day, but for each day that I am alive, I want to spend it with a good quality of life, which is very important to me. My lifestyle allows me to feel good and be active doing the things that I love to do.

These three stories have a few things in common. Each person acknowledged a health concern and initially made small changes in their life to correct it. Linda tried the medication Chantix to help her quit smoking, but it didn't work. Philip began making small changes in his eating and lost fifteen pounds but the weight returned. Judy walked two miles a day, but it wasn't enough for her to keep the weight off. Each person evaluated their situation and decided to make other changes, which led to success. Interestingly, it appeared to be a health threat that served as the catalyst for the changes that finally worked. Linda had a painful pneumonia, which reminded her of her mother's cancer death. Philip's blood pressure was rising and his wife shared her concerns with him. Judy developed painful arthritis. It took time and persistence, but they were ultimately successful with obtaining their goals.

While changing behavior is truly easier said than done, you can do it too. From my perspective, the key ingredients for a longer, better, quality of life involve:

- Increased physical activity. At a minimum, get up and move every hour.
- A diet filled with more fruits and vegetables, low-fat dairy, and lean meats.
- Limiting processed foods, salt, and sugar.
- Reducing alcohol intake.
- Weighing yourself daily and adjusting your lifestyle when weight creeps up.
- Getting a good night's rest.
- Managing your stress triggers. Don't sweat the small stuff.
- Get regular checkups.
- Keep your blood pressure, blood sugar, and cholesterol under control.
- Learn CPR and know what to do in an emergency.
- Have purpose in your life. Keep busy and avoid boredom.
- Use prayer or meditation to calm your restless spirit.
- If you are middle aged with cardiac risk factors, get a non-contrast Coronary Artery Calcium Heart Scan to check for hidden heart disease.

Final Take Away Points

Despite warnings to the contrary, far too many Americans engage in unhealthy behaviors. The magnitude of this problem will have far-reaching consequences for a health care system already burdened by an aging baby boomer population. Therefore, it is imperative that individuals change course and alter harmful behaviors. The length and quality of life will be improved. However, a multitude of barriers impede the best of intentions to live a healthier life. Don't be afraid to seek out the help of a lifestyle consultant and get started making small realistic changes. While changing course is difficult, it can be done and every little change counts. Each step of success will move you down the road toward your goal. You can do it!

I hope that you found this book helpful. If you need additional assistance or resources, please visit my Web site at www.living4ahealthyheart.com. I'm available for individual consulting and public speaking. Finally, please send me an e-mail of your personal lifestyle success stories. God bless you on your individual journey.

Our body is a gift from God.

So, whether you eat or drink, or whatever
you do, do all for the glory of God.

The *Bible*,—1 Corinthians 10:31
(Paul, a follower of Jesus Christ)

About My Services

Lifestyle Consulting for the Public

After reading this book, I hope that you are now ready to make some changes in your life. My approach to lifestyle consulting is based on the latest research into what works to help people overcome barriers. I've counseled hundreds of people to move toward better health. We will work together for simple solutions that will fit more easily into your everyday life. My philosophy is simple, "The best changes are the ones that you aren't aware that you are making." Small changes are more realistic and often lead to positive improvements in your health. If you would like information on lifestyle consulting, risk factors, or answers to your heart-related questions, visit my Web site at www.living4ahealthyheart.com to learn how I work with patients.

Lifestyle Consulting for the Medical Community

Healthcare providers are busy diagnosing cardiovascular disease and treating the risk factors that worsen the problem. Most of you have minimal time to counsel patients on the complicated process of lifestyle change. I'm available to work with your patients to provide lifestyle counseling via telephone. Currently, I am licensed in twenty-six states. You may visit my Web site for a list of the states and how to contact me to work in your state as well. If you would like patient brochures that advertise my services, we would be happy to send you a complimentary patient supply.

Presentations for the Business Community

If you are a business owner concerned with rising health care costs for your employees and you would like to help them eliminate bad habits, my motivational talk may help you: "Wake-Up Call 911: It's Time to Reduce Your Risk for a Heart Attack or Stroke." It is a motivational talk designed to spark an interest in behavior change. Program length and topics are customized to meet the needs of your audience. In addition to heart attack and stroke prevention, some of the other popular programs include: weight loss, portion control, smoking cessation, cholesterol or blood pressure control, pre-diabetes, stress management, or overcoming barriers.

Presentations for the Medical Community

I'm also available to update medical staff on the latest lifestyle counseling techniques that enhance motivation and current information on cardiac risk factors. My expertise in how to utilize the results from a coronary artery calcium heart scan will help you to enhance motivation in your patients as well.

Copies of the Book

If you would like to purchase copies of this book for employees, patients, friends, and family, you may contact my book publisher at www.tatepublishing.com. Complimentary bookmarks that provide information regarding how to purchase copies of this book for employees or patients may be obtained through my Web site as well at www.living4ahealthyheart.com.

God bless you all on your journey toward a healthier life.

About the Author

Professional

Jennie E. Johnson was awarded a PhD in nursing from Loyola University, Chicago, in 2012, a Bachelor of Science in Nursing from Aurora University in 2006, and a Diploma in Nursing from Wichita, St. Joseph School of Nursing in 1974. Dr. Johnson is a registered nurse with a vast experience in caring for cardiovascular patients in critical care and telemetry units. Since 1998, she has been involved with disseminating results and providing lifestyle counseling to patients following a coronary artery calcium heart scan. She is certified in cardiology and served as a Content Expert Panel member for the national Cardiac/Vascular nursing exam. Dr. Johnson is a member of the Preventive Cardiovascular Nurses Association (PCNA), the American College of Cardiology, (ACC), the nursing honor society Sigma Theta Tau, and the American Heart Association (AHA). Her research interests include the impact of the awareness of a coronary artery calcium heart scan on behavior change and understanding the other influences that impact successful lifestyle changes.

She received the 2012 Cardiovascular Disease (CVD) Prevention Graduation Award from PCNA that "demonstrated a strong commitment to the prevention of CVD through excellence in nursing practice or research." Jennie counseled hundreds of patients to make healthier behavior choices and created a variety of highly regarded health related educational programs. Her audiences ranged in age from elementary school children, teenagers, adults, and corporations.

Personal

Jennie and her husband John are co-founders of Living for A Healthy Heart, LLC. They have three married children, a granddaughter and grandson with two babies on the way. The *Bible* verse that guides her life is: "But seek first the kingdom of God and His righteousness, and all these things will be added unto you" (Matthew 6:33). Jennie and John live on a lake in the mountains of Northern Idaho.

Acknowledgments

One year was devoted to the full-time writing of this book. It would not have been possible without the encouragement, wisdom, and financial support of my husband John. You believed in the importance of the work and the need to get it into the hands of at risk Americans. You kept me centered and enforced writing breaks to get me out of the chair to go for a walk. Without you, this book would have never come to fruition. You are the song in my heart.

I am enormously indebted to my oldest daughter and Ear Nose and Throat surgeon, Dr. Katherine Aberle, who served as the primary editor for the book and Web site designer for our business: Living for a Healthy Heart, LLC. Only when it passed your eyes, did I view it ready to go to Tate Publishing. Your medical advice was spot on. Despite your hectic life, you carved out time to help me with these endeavors and finish the book. I will be forever grateful.

Special thanks also to my daughter, Stephanie McCormick, FNP-C, who used her nurse practitioner experience to ensure that patients and clinicians would understand the chapters. Your insight, encouragement and prayer support was tremendously helpful!

My grown children, Katie, Joe, Stephanie and their spouses, remain the stress busters in my life. You have grown into wonderful adults who are adding phenomenal people to our family. Babies Anna and Caleb bring us such joy.

Special thanks to my son and daughter-in-law, Joseph and Charlene Johnson, for posing for the Walk the Dog pictures.

I have been blessed with the love of two mothers. Thanks, Mom (Ilene), for all of those wonderful nursing stories that you shared when I was a little girl. You are the reason why I became a nurse. Thanks to my mother-in-law (Ellen) for your support and encouragement.

A surprising find during this process was the writing abilities of one of my lay reviewers, my brother John. Your edits were unbelievably helpful. I look forward to your book about the colorful characters that you have met while traveling down the road in your RV "down by the river."

I wanted to end the book with lessons from average people who overcame personal barriers and conquered a difficult behavior problem. Special thanks to Linda Schulte, Philip McCormick, and Judy Cox for sharing your stories.

For this book, I asked a few nonmedical persons to read various chapters and provide feedback. The team ranged from thirty to eighty-four years in age, with careers that varied from a bank teller to an individual with a PhD in engineering. Although I wrote this book in a language that patients should understand, it was interesting to note the areas that needed further clarification. Their insight helped to shed light on misconceptions and made this book more relevant for patients. Thank you: George Ott, Philip McCormick, Joseph Johnson, Ellen Johnson, Jerry and Jan Melberg. Special thanks to Lori Johnson, Neil Oliver, and Pastor Neil Bloom for reading the completed work.

Early in the development of this book, I was blessed with excellent mentoring provided by best-selling authors and national professional speakers Debra Benton and LeAnn Thieman. Debra has written several books on executive coaching and provided invaluable insight regarding the publishing and marketing of a book. Her skills as the "CEO Whisperer" not only improve professionalism for success within the corporate workplace but also in life as well. LeAnn co-authored *Chicken Soup for the Nurse's Soul*. She is a nursing hero who airlifted one hundred orphan babies from Vietnam at the end of the war. Both of you provided suggestions and guidance that were immeasurably appreciated.

Professionally, I would like to thank the following healthcare providers who reviewed various segments in the book: pharmacist Mark Jobst, RPh (pharmaceutical sections), nurse practitioners Jacque McKernan, RN, PhD (diabetes), and Kathleen Zarling, MS, RN, ACNS- BC (smoking), Michael Burke, MD (smoking), and dentists David Carlson, DDS and Michael Trantow, DDS (periodontal disease section). Your insight was invaluable.

I wish to thank the leaders of the Preventive Cardiovascular Nurses Association (PCNA) for your encouragement, support, and marketing of the book. Special thanks to Lynne Braun, PhD, CNP for reviewing the book. Dr. Braun is a national nursing leader and frequent speaker for PCNA events. Your edits were extremely helpful. My membership in PCNA remains a powerful resource. The conventions and educational opportunities have been most helpful in keeping me up-to-date on the latest changes within our specialty. The American College of Cardiology updates were helpful to keep the book current as well.

Throughout one's education journey, we are exposed to teachers who profoundly enhance how we think about things. I will never forget Mr. Witherspoon from fifth grade. In writing this book, one professor's words kept ringing through my ears: Meg Gulanick, PhD, APRN from Loyola University in Chicago, Illinois. Dr. Gulanick encouraged and supported my efforts to go back to school and served as my dissertation chair. I wish to thank her for excellent leadership, passion for the prevention of cardiovascular disease, and tireless support of me throughout the dissertation research project. You were in my head as I wrote this book. Thank you also for your thoughtful edits of the book. Other Loyola nursing faculty that helped me grow in my role as a nursing researcher were Dr. Sue Penckofer (diabetes, depression, and Vitamin D studies) and Dr. Linda Janusek (stress and breast cancer studies).

Several physicians read the entire book and provided enthusiastic support and insight. Thank you so much: Stephen DeVries, MD, Donald Chisholm, MD, and Vincent Bufalino, MD, and dentists Michael Trantow, DDS, and David Carlson, DDS. Cardiologist Dr. Vincent Bufalino was the visionary who brought the coronary artery calcium heart scan technology to Naperville, Illinois. He wanted cardiac staff nurses to disseminate the results and review lifestyle options with patients. It was in this role that my passion for lifestyle counseling and public speaking was ignited.

I was especially honored by the support of world, renowned psychologists Brain Wansink, PH.D *(Mindless Eating)*, and James Prochaska, PH.D *(Stages of Change Theory)*. Both of you have contributed so much to our understanding of the motivations involved with changing behavior. I only hope that I translated your work in a manner that helps other healthcare practitioners utilize your invaluable information within the clinical setting.

Thank you to the team at Tate Publishing for their work in the production of this book.

Some of the proceeds from the sale of this book will be donated to the Preventive Cardiovascular Nurses Association, the American Heart Association, and various Christian charities in support of their wonderful work to help others.

Finally, my father died suddenly at forty-six years old from a massive heart attack when I was a young nurse just starting my career in a coronary care unit in Seattle, Washington. His death was a shock for all of us. I buried his memory and all of his stories for many years. In an ethics course at Loyola, we were asked to bring a picture and share something that had a profound impact on our life. I pulled out the image of my dad walking my sister down the wedding aisle five days before he died. It was only then that I realized that my whole nursing career has been devoted to preventing similar fates for other families. It is in the memory of my Dad (Murph), that this book was written. I am most thankful for the gift of writing and all other blessings that God has showered upon me. May the words within this book be a blessing of health for you and your family as well.

Appendix

Healthy Weight and Overweight BMI Classes

BMI Ht	19	20	21	22	23	24	25	26	27	28	29
4'10"	91	96	100	105	110	115	119	124	129	134	138
4'11"	94	99	104	109	114	119	124	128	133	138	143
5'	97	102	107	112	118	123	128	133	138	143	148
5'1"	100	106	111	116	122	127	132	137	143	148	153
5'2"	104	109	115	120	126	131	136	142	147	153	158
5'3"	107	113	118	124	130	135	141	146	152	158	163
5'4"	110	116	122	128	134	140	145	151	157	163	169
5'5"	114	120	126	132	138	144	150	156	162	168	174
5'6"	118	124	130	136	142	148	155	161	167	173	179
5'7"	121	127	134	140	146	153	159	166	172	178	185
5'8"	125	131	138	144	151	158	164	171	177	184	190
5'9"	128	135	142	149	155	162	169	176	182	189	196
5'10"	132	139	146	153	160	167	174	181	188	195	202
5'11"	136	143	150	157	165	172	179	186	193	200	208
6'	140	147	154	162	169	177	184	191	199	206	213
6'1"	144	151	159	166	174	182	189	197	204	212	219
6'2"	148	155	163	171	179	186	194	202	210	218	225
6'3"	152	160	168	176	184	192	200	208	216	224	232
6'4"	156	164	172	180	189	197	205	213	221	230	238
Healthy Weight							**Overweight**				

* Preventive Cardiovascular Nurses Association (PCNA)

*Adapted from the Evidence Report of Clinical Guidelines on the Identification, Evaluation, and Treatment of Overweight and Obesity in Adults, 1998. *NIH/National Heart, Lung, and Blood Institute (NHLBI)*

Obese BMI Class I and II

BMI	30	31	32	33	34	35	36	37	38	39
Ht										
4'10"	143	148	153	158	162	167	172	177	181	186
4'11"	148	153	158	163	168	173	178	183	188	193
5'	153	158	163	168	174	179	184	189	194	199
5'1"	158	164	169	174	180	185	190	195	201	206
5'2"	164	169	175	180	186	191	196	202	207	213
5'3"	169	175	180	186	191	197	203	208	214	220
5'4"	174	180	186	192	197	204	209	215	221	227
5'5"	180	186	192	198	204	210	216	222	228	234
5'6"	186	192	198	204	210	216	223	229	235	241
5'7"	191	198	204	211	217	223	230	236	242	249
5'8"	197	203	210	216	223	230	236	243	249	256
5'9"	203	209	216	223	230	236	243	250	257	263
5'10"	209	216	222	229	236	243	250	257	264	271
5'11"	215	222	229	236	243	250	257	265	272	279
6'	221	228	235	242	250	258	265	272	279	287
6'1"	227	235	242	250	257	265	272	280	288	295
6'2"	233	241	249	256	264	272	280	287	295	303
6'3"	240	248	256	264	272	279	287	295	303	311
6'4"	246	254	263	271	279	287	295	304	312	320
Obese Class I					**Obese Class II**					

* Preventive Cardiovascular Nurses Association (PCNA)

*Adapted from Evidence Report of Clinical Guidelines on the Identification, Evaluation, and Treatment of Overweight and Obesity in Adults, 1998. *NIH/National Heart, Lung, and Blood Institute (NHLBI)*

Obese BMI Class III

BMI Ht.	40	41	42	43	44	45	46	47	48	49	50	51
4'10"	191	196	201	205	210	215	220	224	229	234	239	244
4'11"	198	203	208	212	217	222	227	232	237	242	247	252
5'	204	209	215	220	225	230	235	240	245	250	255	261
5'1"	211	217	222	227	232	238	243	248	254	259	264	269
5'2"	218	224	229	235	240	246	251	256	262	267	273	278
5'3"	225	231	237	242	248	254	259	265	270	278	282	287
5'4"	232	238	244	250	256	262	267	273	279	285	291	296
5'5"	240	246	252	258	264	270	276	282	288	294	300	306
5'6"	247	253	260	266	272	278	284	291	297	303	309	315
5'7"	255	261	268	274	280	287	293	299	306	312	319	325
5'8"	262	269	276	282	289	295	302	308	315	322	328	335
5'9"	270	277	284	291	297	304	311	318	324	331	338	345
5'10"	278	285	292	299	306	313	320	327	334	341	348	355
5'11"	286	293	301	308	315	322	329	338	343	351	358	365
6'	294	302	309	316	324	331	338	346	353	361	368	375
6'1"	302	310	318	325	333	340	348	355	363	371	378	386
6'2"	311	319	326	334	342	350	358	365	373	381	389	396
6'3"	319	327	335	343	351	359	367	375	383	391	399	407
6'4"	328	336	344	353	361	369	377	385	394	402	410	418

Obese Class III

* Preventive Cardiovascular Nurses Association (PCNA)

*Adapted from Evidence Report of Clinical Guidelines on the Identification, Evaluation, and Treatment of Overweight and Obesity in Adults, 1998. *NIH/National Heart, Lung, and Blood Institute (NHLBI)*

Strategies to Help You Quit Tobacco Use

Make a list of your reasons for quitting and a list of potential barriers.
Call a smoking hotline to learn how to quit your particular habit.
Speak with your healthcare provider about smoking cessation medications.
Set a quit date for 2 weeks. No tobacco after this date!
During this two week period before you quit, try smoking with the other hand. If you smoke while you sit, stand. Change your habits to prepare you for your quit date.
"Morning": drink tea instead of coffee. Change your usual routine.
Remove tobacco products from your home, car and all other places
Tell your support team and peer tobacco users that you are quitting.
Develop a plan for stressful situations.
Encourage others "not" to smoke around you, which may trigger cravings.
"Quite date": Keep busy, get your rest, eat regular meals, snack on healthy foods.
Suck on cinnamon candy, which may make any tobacco product taste terrible.
Carry a pen that you can click on and off in your hands when you feel anxious.
Get your teeth cleaned.
Avoid alcohol, which may lead to relapse.
Remember cravings are like a woman in labor, they peak within a few minutes then go away. Be ready with a nicotine replacement medication.
You will miss the enjoyment of smoking due to the loss of nicotine. Don't be sabotaged by this reaction.
If you relapse TRY AGAIN! Even using tobacco one time may trigger your addiction.
Stay positive…reward yourself for getting through the first 3 days, first week, first 2 weeks, etc. Use the money you are saving for a special reward.
Your health is improving. You look better and you don't have smoker's breath.
Keep your list of benefits for quitting in a place where you can see them everyday.
Quitting tobacco use will be one of the hardest things that you have ever done but you can do it!
*Treating Tobacco Use and Dependence *U.S. Department of Health and Human Services*

Determining Your Target Heart Rate (THR)

Calculating Target Heart Rate Range Using the Karvonen Method
Calculate your resting heart rate (HR resting) by sitting for 10 minutes and then taking your pulse: _____
Calculate your maximum heart rate (HR max) by subtracting your age from 220. _____
Next select how hard you want to exercise [a range between 40% (.40) and 85% (.85)]. This intensity is based on your maximum heart rate. Note: Fit persons will have higher intensity ranges while less fit persons will begin with lower ranges. Patients on beta-blocker medications can also use this formula.
Formula for Target Heart Rate Ranges =   **[(HR max – HR rest) X % low intensity goal] + HR rest = low pulse rate range =_____**
[(HR max – HR rest) X % high intensity goal] + HR rest = high pulse rate range =_____
Example: 45 year old sedentary obese man who has permission to begin a program.   Maximum heart rate (HR max) = 220 – 45 = 175   Resting pulse rate (HR resting) = 75   Target Heart Rate for lowest intensity of 40% = [(175-75) X .40] + 75 =115   Target Heart Rate for highest intensity of 60% = [(175-75) X .60] + 75 = 135   **Thus the exercising target heart rate range is between 115 and 135.**   As his fitness improves his target heart rate ranges may be adjusted as well.
*Adapted from the *American College of Sport's Medicine Guidelines for Exercise Testing and Prescription, 2006*

Heat Index Table

NOAA's National Weather Service

Heat Index
Temperature (°F)

Relative Humidity (%)	80	82	84	86	88	90	92	94	96	98	100	102	104	106	108	110
40	80	81	83	85	88	91	94	97	101	105	109	114	119	124	130	136
45	80	82	84	87	89	93	96	100	104	109	114	119	124	130	137	
50	81	83	85	88	91	95	99	103	108	113	118	124	131	137		
55	81	84	86	89	93	97	101	106	112	117	124	130	137			
60	82	84	88	91	95	100	105	110	116	123	129	137				
65	82	85	89	93	98	103	108	114	121	128	136					
70	83	86	90	95	100	105	112	119	126	134						
75	84	88	92	97	103	109	116	124	132							
80	84	89	94	100	106	113	121	129								
85	85	90	96	102	110	117	126	135								
90	86	91	98	105	113	122	131									
95	86	93	100	108	117	127										
100	87	95	103	112	121	132										

Likelihood of Heat Disorders with Prolonged Exposure or Strenuous Activity

☐ Caution   ☐ Extreme Caution   ▨ Danger   ■ Extreme Danger

Cold Wind Chill Index

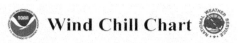

Wind Chill Chart

		Temperature (°F)																
Calm	**40**	**35**	**30**	**25**	**20**	**15**	**10**	**5**	**0**	**-5**	**-10**	**-15**	**-20**	**-25**	**-30**	**-35**	**-40**	**-45**
5	36	31	25	19	13	7	1	-5	-11	-16	-22	-28	-34	-40	-46	-52	-57	-63
10	34	27	21	15	9	3	-4	-10	-16	-22	-28	-35	-41	-47	-53	-59	-66	-72
15	32	25	19	13	6	0	-7	-13	-19	-26	-32	-39	-45	-51	-58	-64	-71	-77
20	30	24	17	11	4	-2	-9	-15	-22	-29	-35	-42	-48	-55	-61	-68	-74	-81
25	29	23	16	9	3	-4	-11	-17	-24	-31	-37	-44	-51	-58	-64	-71	-78	-84
30	28	22	15	8	1	-5	-12	-19	-26	-33	-39	-46	-53	-60	-67	-73	-80	-87
35	28	21	14	7	0	-7	-14	-21	-27	-34	-41	-48	-55	-62	-69	-76	-82	-89
40	27	20	13	6	-1	-8	-15	-22	-29	-36	-43	-50	-57	-64	-71	-78	-84	-91
45	26	19	12	5	-2	-9	-16	-23	-30	-37	-44	-51	-58	-65	-72	-79	-86	-93
50	26	19	12	4	-3	-10	-17	-24	-31	-38	-45	-52	-60	-67	-74	-81	-88	-95
55	25	18	11	4	-3	-11	-18	-25	-32	-39	-46	-54	-61	-68	-75	-82	-89	-97
60	25	17	10	3	-4	-11	-19	-26	-33	-40	-48	-55	-62	-69	-76	-84	-91	-98

Wind (mph)

Frostbite Times ■ 30 minutes ■ 10 minutes ■ 5 minutes

Wind Chill (°F) = 35.74 + 0.6215T - 35.75(V$^{0.16}$) + 0.4275T(V$^{0.16}$)

Where, T= Air Temperatur· (°F) V= Wind Speed (mph)

Effective 11/01/01

National Weather Service (NOAA)

Air Quality Index

0-50	Good	Green	Air quality is considered satisfactory, and air pollution poses little or no risk.
51-100	Moderate	Yellow	Air quality is acceptable; however, for some pollutants there may be a moderate health concern for a very small number of people who are unusually sensitive to air pollution.
101-150	Unhealthy for Sensitive Groups	Orange	Members of sensitive groups may experience health effects. The general public is not likely to be affected.
151-200	Unhealthy	Red	Everyone may begin to experience health effects; members of sensitive groups may experience more serious health effects.
201-300	Very Unhealthy	Purple	Health warnings of emergency conditions. The entire population is more likely to be affected.
301-500	Hazardous	Maroon	Health alert; everyone may experience more serious health effects.
* Air Quality Index (AQI)-A Guide to Air Quality and Your Health			

Reference

Introduction: Who Should Read This Book

1. Brian Wansink, *Mindless Eating: Why We Eat More Than We Think* (New York, NY: Bantam Dell, 2007):13.

Heart Attack and Stroke Basics

1. "Taber's Cyclopedic Medical Dictionary," *Tabers Online*, 2013/accessed August 3, 2014. http://www.tabers.com/tabe rsonline?svar=a%7cgoandsvar=c%7ctpdaandgclid=CJqo2Kz YtLgCFe1_Qgod6GQASg.
2. "Warning Signs of a Heart Attack," *American Heart Association*, 2012/accessed August 3, 2014. http://www. heart.org/HEARTORG/Conditions/HeartAttack/Warning Signso faHeartAttack/Warning-Signs-of-a-Heart-Attack_ UCM_002039_Article.jsp.
3. *Guidelines for Cardiac Rehabilitation and Secondary Prevention Programs (5th. ed)*. (Champaign, IL: Human Kinetics Publishers, 2013).
4. "Stroke Warning Signs and Symptoms," *American Stroke Association*, 2013/accessed August 3, 2014. http://stroke

association.org/STROKEORG/WarningSigns/Stroke-Warning-Signs-%09and-Symptoms_UCM_308528_Sub HomePage.jsp.

5. George Spratto and Adrienne Woods, *Delmar Nurse's Drug Handbook* (Clifton Park, NY: Delmar Cengage Learning, 2013).

6. Alan Go, Dariush Mozaffarin, Veronique Roger, Emelia Benjamin, Jarett Berry, Michael Blaha et al., "AHA Statistical Update: Heart Disease and Stroke Statistics-2014," *Circulation* 129 (2014), December 18, 2014/acessed August 2, 2014. http://circ.ahajournals.org/content/early/2013/12/18/01. cir.0000441139.02102.80.

7. Michael Fiesbein, and Robert Siegel, "How Big Are Atherosclerotic Plaques that Rupture?" *Circulation* 94 (1996): 2662–2666/accessed August 3, 2014. http://circ. ahajournals.org/content/94/10/2662.full doi:10.1161/01. CIR.94.10.2662.

Are You At Risk?

1. Alan Go, Dariush Mozaffarin, Veronique Roger, Emelia Benjamin, Jarett Berry, Michael Blaha et al., "AHA Statistical Update: Heart Disease and Stroke Statistics-2014," *Circulation* 129 (2014), December 18, 2014/acessed August 2, 2014. http://circ.ahajournals.org/content/early/2013/12/18/01.cir. 0000441139.02102.80.

2. "What Are the Key Statistics about Prostate Cancer?" *American Cancer Society* (2014)/accessed August 3, 2014. http://www.cancer.org/cancer/prostatecancer/detailedguide/ prostate-cancer-key-statistics.

3. "Men and Heart Disease Fact Sheet," *Centers for Disease Control* (2013)/accessed August 3, 2014. http://www.cdc. gov/dhdsp/data_statistics/fact_sheets/fs_men_heart.htm.

4. Irwin Rosenstock, "What Research in Motivation Suggests for Public Health," *American Journal of Public Health* 50 (1960): 295–302.

5. "Framingham Heart Study," 2014/accessed August 3, 2014. http://www.framinghamheartstudy.org/about-fhs/history.php.

6. Leslie Moore, Laura Kimble, and Ptlene Minick, "Perceptions of Cardiac Risk Factors and Risk-reduction Behavior in Women with Known Coronary Heart Disease," *Journal of Cardiovascular Nursing* 25 no. 6 (2010): 433–443/ accessed August 3, 2014. http://www.ncbi.nlm.nih.gov/pubmed/20938247.

7. Neil Stone, Jennifer Robinson, Alice Lichtenstein, Noel Merz, Conrad Blum, Robert Eckel et al. "2013 ACC/AHA Guideline on the Treatment of Blood Cholesterol to Reduce Atherosclerotic Cardiovascular Risk in Adults: A Third Report of the American College of Cardiology/American Heart Association Task Force on Practice Guidelines," *Circulation* (2013)/ accessed August 3, 2014. http://circ.ahajournals.org/content/early/2013/11/11/01.cir.0000437738.63853.7a.

8. William Fearon, "Is a Myocardial Infarction More Likely to Result from a Mild Coronary Lesion or an Ischemia-Producing One?" *Circulation Interventions* (2011)/accessed August 3, 2014. http://circinterventions.ahajournals.org/content/4/6/539.full.pdf+html.

9. Matthew Budoff, Stephen Achenbach, Roger Blumenthal, Jeffrey Carr, Jonathan Goldin, Philip Greenland et al. "Assessment of Coronary Artery Disease by Cardiac Computed Tomography: A Scientific Statement from the American Heart Association Committee on Cardiovascular Imaging and Intervention, Council on Cardiovascular Radiology and Intervention, and Committee on Cardiac Imaging, Council on Clinical Cardiology," *Circulation* 114

(2006), 1761–1791/accessed August 3, 2014. http://circ.ahajournals.org/content/114/16/1761.full.

10. Khurram Nasir, Leslee Shaw, Matthew Budoff, Paul Ridker and Jessica Pena, "Coronary Artery Calcium Scanning Should Be Used for Primary Prevention," *Journal of the College of Cardiology* 5 no. 1 (2012): 111–118. DOI: 10.1016/j.jcmg.2011.11.007/accessed September 1, 2014. http://imaging.onlinejacc.org/article.aspx?articleid=1097059.

11. Rameu Meneghelo, Raul Santos, Breno Almeida, Jairo Hidal, Tania Martinex, Reno Moron et al., "Distribution of Coronary Artery Calcium Scores Determined by Ultrafast Computed Tomography in 2.253 Asymptomatic White Men," *Arq Bras Cardiol* 81 no. suppl. 7 (2003): 32–36./accessed August 3, 2014. http://www.scielo.br/pdf/abc/v81s7/en_a03v81s7.pdf.

12. Philip Greenland, Robert Bonow, Bruce Brundage, Matthew Budoff, Mark Eisenberg et al., "ACC/AHA 2007 Clinical Expert Consensus Document on Coronary Artery Calcium Scoring by Computed Tomography in Global Cardiovascular Risk Assessment and in Evaluation of Patients with Chest Pain," *Circulation* 115 (2007): 402–426/accessed August 3, 2014. http://circ.ahajournals.org/content/115/3/402.full.pdf+html.

13. David Goff, Donald Lloyd-Jones, Glen Bennett, Sean Coady, Ralph D'Agostino, Raymond Gibbons et al. "2013 ACC/AHA Guideline on the Assessment of Cardiovascular Risk: A Report of the American College of Cardiology/American Heart Association Task Force on Practice Guidelines," *Circulation*, (2013) August 3, 2014/accessed February 28, 2104. http://circ.ahajournals.org/content/early/2013/11/11/01.cir.0000437741.48606.98.

14. Scan Directory.com (2007)/accessed August 3, 2014. http://www.scandirectory.com/content/calcium_scan.asp.

15. Arthur Agatston, *The South Beach Heart Program: The 4–Step Plan that Can Save Your Life*, (New York, NY: Holtzbrinck Publishers, (2007): 217.

16. Jorg Hausleiter, Tanja Meyer, Franziska Hermann, Martin Hadamitzky, Markus Krebs, Thomas Gerber et al., "Estimated Radiation Dose Associated with Cardiac CT Angiography," *Journal of the American Medical Association* 301 no. 5 (2009): 500–507/accessed August 3, 2014. http://www.ncbi.nlm.nih. gov/pubmed/19190314.

17. Lawrence Altman, "The Doctors World; James Fixx: the Enigma of Heart Disease," *The Doctors World*, July 24, 1984/accessed August 3, 2014. http://www.nytimes. com/1984/07/24/science/the-doctor-s-world-james-fixx-the-enigma-of-heart-disease.html.

18. "James Gandolfini Did Not Die of Natural Causes," *Huffington Celebrity*, June 6, 2013/accessed August 3, 2014. http://www.huffingtonpost.com/neal-barnard-md/james-gandolfini-did-not-_b_3491047.html.

19. Tom Gliatto, "In a Heartbeat," *People*, January 31, 2000/ accessed August 3, 2014 http://www.people.com/people/archive/article/0,,20130377,00.html.

20. Loren Grush, "George Bush's Artery Was 95 Percent Blocked, Source Says," *Fox News*, October 15, 2013/accessed February 25, 2014. http://www.foxnews.com/health/2013/10/15/george-w-bush-artery-was-5–percent-blocked-source-says/.

21. Billy Hallowell, "TV Producer and Host Dick Clark Dies after Massive Heart Attack," *Entertainment*. April 18, 2012/ accessed February 25, 2014. http://www.theblaze. com/stories/2012/04/18/famed-television-producer-dick-clark-has-died/.

22. "Have You Got 'Sharon Stone Syndrome'?" *MailOnline*/ accessed February 25, 2014. http://www.dailymail.co.uk/health/article-86282/Have-got-Sharon- Stone- Syndrome.html.

23. Wenn, "Stone Speaks of Stroke Horror," *Contactmusic. com*, August 10, 2004/accessed August 3, 2014. http:// www.contactmusic.com/news-article/stone-speaks-of-m stroke-horror.

Cholesterol: The Good, the Bad, End the Confusion

1. Alan Go, Dariush Mozaffarin, Veronique Roger, Emelia Benjamin, Jarett Berry, Michael Blaha et al., "AHA Statistical Update: Heart Disease and Stroke Statistics-2014," *Circulation* 129 (2014), December 18, 2014/acessed August 2, 2014. http://circ.ahajournals.org/content/early/2013/12/18/01. cir.0000441139.02102.80.
2. Elizabeth Arias, "United States Life Tables, 2003," *National Vital Statistics Reports* 62 no. 7 (2007)/accessed October 17, 2014. http://www.cdc.gov/nchs/data/nvsr/nvsr62/nvsr 62_07.pdf.
3. National Cholesterol Education Program (NCEP) "Executive Summary of the Third Report of the National Cholesterol Education Program (NCEP) Expert Panel on Detection, Evaluation, and Treatment of High Blood Cholesterol in Adults (Adult Treatment Panel III)," *U.S. Department of Health and Human Services*. NIH Publication No. 01–3670, (2001).
4. Scott Grundy, James Cleeman, Stephen Daniels, Karen Donato, Robert Eckel, Barry Franklin et al. "Diagnosis and Management of the Metabolic Syndrome: An American Heart Association/National Heart, Lung, and Blood Institute Scientific Statement. Executive Summary," *Circulation* 112 no. 17 (2005): 2735–2752/ accessed August 3, 2014. http:// circ.ahajournals.org/content/112/17/2735.full.pdf+html.
5. Neil Stone, Jennifer Robinson, Alice Lichtenstein, Noel Merz, Conrad Blum, Robert Eckel et al. "2013 ACC/AHA Guideline on the Treatment of Blood Cholesterol to Reduce

Atherosclerotic Cardiovascular Risk in Adults: A Third Report of the American College of Cardiology/American Heart Association Task Force on Practice Guidelines," *Circulation* (2013)/accessed August 3, 2014. http://circ.ahajournals.org/content/early/2013/11/11/01.cir.0000437738.63853.7a.

6. Amit Sachdeva, Christopher Cannon, Prakash Deedwania, Kenneth LaBresh, Sidney Smith, David Dai et al., "Lipid Levels in Patients Hospitalized with Coronary Artery Disease: An Analysis of 136,905 Hospitalizations in Get With the Guidelines," *American Heart Journal* 157 no. 1 (2009)/ accessed August 3, 2014. http://www.ahjonline.com/article/S0002–8703(08)00717–5/abstract.

7. *Step By Step: Eating to Lower Your Blood Cholesterol, US Department of Health and Human Services*, (NIH Publication No. 98–2920, 1998).

8. "Saturated Fats," *American Heart Association* (2013)/accessed August 3, 2014. http://www.heart.org/HEARTORG/GettingHealthy/FatsAndOils/Fats101/Saturated-Fats_UCM_301110_Article.jsp.

9. "Knowing Your Fats," *American Heart Association* (2013)/accessed August 3, 2014. http://www.heart.org/HEARTORG/GettingHealthy/NutritionCenter/Knowing-Your-Fats_UCM_305976_Article.jsp.

10. "Fish and Omega-3 Fatty Acids," *American Heart Association* (2013)/accessed August 3, 2014. http://www.heart.org/HEARTORG/GettingHealthy/NutritionCenter/HealthyDietGoals/Fish-and-Omega-3–Fatty-Acids_UCM_303248_Article.jsp.

11. George Spratto and Adrienne Woods, *Delmar Nurse's Drug Handbook* (Clifton Park, NY: Delmar Cengage Learning, 2013).

12. "FDA: Limit Use of 80 mg Simvastatin," *Department of Health and Human Services*, June 8, 2011/accessed August 3,

2014. http://www.fda.gov/forconsumers/consumerupdates/ucm257884.htm.

13. Stephen Devries and Winifred Conkling, *What Your Doctor May Not Tell You About Cholesterol: The Latest Natural Treatments and Scientific Advances in One Breakthrough Program*, (New York, NY:A Lynd Sonberg Book Wellness Central, 2007), 26.

High Blood Pressure: The Silent Killer

1. Alan Go, Dariush Mozaffarin, Veronique Roger, Emelia Benjamin, Jarett Berry, William Borden et al., "AHA Statistical Update: Heart Disease and Stroke Statistics-2013," *Circulation* 127 (2013): e110/accessed August 7, 2014. http://circ.ahajournals.org/content/127/1/e6.full.pdf+html.

2. Aram Chobanian, George Bakris, Henry Black, William Cushman, Lee Green, Joseph Izzo et al. "The Seventh Report of the Joint National Committee on Prevention, Detection, Evaluation, and Treatment of High Blood Pressure: The JNC 7 Report," *JAMA* 289, no. 19(2003): 2560–2572/accessed August 7, 2014. http://www.nhlbi.nih.gov/guidelines/hypertension/jnc7full.pdf.

3. Carol Taylor, Carol Lillis and Priscilla LeMone, *Fundamentals of Nursing: The Art and Science of Nursing Care (5th ed.)*, (New York, NY: Lipincott Williams and Wilkins, 2005), 525.

4. James Paul, Suzanne Oparil, Barry Carter, William Cushman, Cheryl Dennison- Himmelfarb, Joel Handler et al. "2014 Evidence-based Guideline for the Management of High Blood Pressure in Adults Report from the Panel Members Appointed to the Eight Joint National Committee (JNC 8)," *Journal of the American Medical Association*, December 18, 2013/accessed August 7, 2014. http://jama.jamanetwork.com/article.aspx?articleid=1791497. Doi:10.1001/jama.2013.284427.

5. "High Blood Pressure During Pregnancy," *National Institute of Health, National Heart Lung and Blood Institute*/accessed October 17, 2014. http://www.nhlbi.nih.gov/health/resources/heart/hbp-pregnancy.htm.

6. Thomas Pickering and William White. "Position Paper: ASH Position Paper: Home and Ambulatory Blood Pressure Monitoring When and How to Use Self (Home) and Ambulatory Blood Pressure Monitoring," *Journal of Clinical Hypertension 10, no. 11 (2008): 850–855/* accessed August 7, 2014. http://onlinelibrary.wiley.com/doi/10.1111/j.1751–7176.2008.00043.x/full.

7. Thomas Pickering, Nancy Houston Miller, Gbenga Ogedegbe, Lawrence Krakoff, Nancy Artinian and David Geoff. "Call to Action on Use and Reimbursement for Home Blood Pressure Monitoring: Executive Summary: A Joint Scientific Statement for the American Heart Association, American Society of Hypertension and Preventive Cardiovascular Nurses Association," *Hypertension* 52, no. 1 (2008):1–9/ accessed August 7, 2014. http://hyper.ahajournals.org/content/52/1/1.full.

8. "Blood Pressure: How Do You Measure Up"? *Preventive Cardiovascular Nurses Association*, (2012)/accessed August 7, 2014. http://pcna.net/patients/blood-m pressure.

9. Robert Eckel, John Jakicic, Jamy Ard, Van Hubbard, Janet de Jesus, I-Min Lee, Alice Lichtenstein et al., "2013 AHA/ACC Guidelines on Lifestyle Management to Reduce Cardiovascular Risk: A Report of the American College of Cardiology/American Heart Association Task Force on Practice Guidelines," *Circulation*, November 12, 2013/ accessed September 9, 2014, http://circ.ahajournals.org/content/early/2013/11/11/01.cir.0000437740.48606.d1.

10. Darwin Labarthe, "Sodium Restriction: Facts and Fiction," *Division for Heart and Stroke Prevention, National Center for Chronic Disease Prevention and Health Promotion and*

Centers for Disease Control and Prevention, 2011)/accessed August 7, 2014. http://www.cdc.gov/cdcgrandrounds/pdf/phgrsodred5final.pdf.

11. *Step By Step: Eating to Lower Your Blood Cholesterol,* US Department of Health and Human Services, NIH Publication No. 98–2920, 1998.

12. "Tim's Cascade Snacks," 2012/accessed August 7, 2014. http://timschips.com/index.php/details/TIMPC#Original%20 Flavor.

13. Lawrence Appel, Thomas Moore, Eva Obarzanek, William Vollmer, Laura Svetkey, Frank Sacks et al. "A Clinical Trial of the Effects of Dietary Patterns on Blood Pressure," *New England Journal of Medicine* 336, no 16 (1997): 1117–1124/accessed August 7, 2014. http://www.nejm.org/doi/full/10.1056/NEJM199704173361601.

14. Lori Smolin and Mary Grosvenor, *Eating Right: An Introduction to Human Nutrition: Nutrition and Weight Management* (Chelsea House: New York, NY, 2005), 29.

15. Junxiu Liu, Xuemei Sui, Carl Lavie, James Hebert, Conrad Earnest, Jiajia Zhang and Steven Blair, "Association of Coffee Consumption with All-cause and Cardiovascular Disease Mortality," *Mayo Clinic,* 2013/accessed August 7, 2014. http://www.mayoclinicproceedings.org/article/S0025–6196(13)00578–8/abstract.

16. "Caffeine Content of Food and Drugs," *Center for Science in the Public Interest,* 2005/accessed August 7, 2014. http://www.cspinet.org/new/cafchart.htm.

17. Ron Rutti, "FDA Warns Against Use of Caffeine Powder that Caused the Death of Lorain County Teen," *The Plain Dealer,* July 19, 2014/accessed August 7, 2014. http://www.cleveland.com/metro/index.ssf/2014/07/fda_warns_against_use_of_ca ffe.htm l.

18. George Spratto and Adrienne Woods, *Delmar Nurse's Drug Handbook*, (Clifton Park, NY: Delmar Cengage Learning, 2013).

19. Carol Cooke, "Take As Directed: A Prescription Not Followed: New Survey Shows Improper Medication Use Reaching Crisis Proportions," *National Community Pharmacists Association*, December 15, 2006/accessed March 6, 2014. http://www.ncpanet.org/pdf/adherence/patientad herence-pr1206.pdf.

20. Joshua Benner, Robert Glynn, Helen Morgun, Peter Neumann, Milton Weinstein and Jerry Avorn, "Long-term Persistence in Use of Statin Therapy in Elderly Patients," *Journal of the American Medical Association*, July 24/31, 2002. http://jama.jamanetwork.com/article.aspx?articleid=195142.

The Danger from Diabetes

1. Alan Go, Dariush Mozaffarin, Veronique Roger, Emelia Benjamin, Jarett Berry, Michael Blaha et al., "AHA Statistical Update: Heart Disease and Stroke Statistics-2014," *Circulation* 129 (2014): e118, December 18, 2014/accessed August 2, 2014. http://circ.ahajournals.org/content/early/2013/12/18/01.cir.0000441139.02102.80.

2. "Statistics About Diabetes: Overall Numbers, Diabetes, and Prediabetes" *American Diabetes Association*, June 10, 2014/accessed October 18, 2014. http://www.diabetes.org/diabetes-basics/statistics/.

3. "American Diabetes Association. Executive Summary: Standards of Medical Care in Diabetes-2013," *Diabetes Care*, January 1, 2013./accessed August 2, 2014. http://care.diabetesjournals.org/content/36/Supplement_1/S4.full.pdf+htm l.

4. National Cholesterol Education Program (NCEP) "Executive Summary of the Third Report of the National Cholesterol

Education Program (NCEP) Expert Panel on Detection, Evaluation, and Treatment of High Blood Cholesterol in Adults (Adult Treatment Panel III)," *U.S. Department of Health and Human Services.* NIH Publication No. 01–3670, (2001).

5. Trevor Orchard, Marinella Temprosa, Ronald Goldberg, Steven Huffnew, Robert Ratner, Santica Maccovina et al. "The Effect of Metformin and Intensive Lifestyle Intervention on the Metabolic Syndrome. The Diabetes Prevention Program Randomized Trial," *Annals of Internal Medicine*, August 19, 2005./accessed August 3, 2014. http://www.ncbi.nlm.nih.gov/pubmed/15838067.

6. George Spratto and Adrienne Woods, *Delmar Nurse's Drug Handbook*, (Clifton Park, NY: Delmar Cengage Learning, 2013).

7. "DKA (Ketoacidosis) and Ketones," *American Diabetes Association*, March 12, 2014/accessed August 3, 2014. http://www.diabetes.org/living-with-diabetes/complications/keto acidosis-dka.html.

8. Mary Marcus, "Mary Tyler Moore Tells How She Took Control of Diabetes," *USA Today*, March 25, 2009/accessed August 3, 2014, http://usatoday30.usatoday.com/life/people/2009–03–22–mtm- diabetes_N.htm.

9. "Cutler Has Learned How to Deal with Diabetes," *ESPN.COM: Chicago Bears*, November 5, 2012/accessed August 3, 2014. http://espn.go.com/blog/chicago/bears/print?id=4679925.

10. "Halley Berry: My Battle with Diabetes," *Mailonline/* accessed August 3, 2014. http://www.dailymail.co.uk/health/article-371528/Halle-Berry-My-battle- diabetes.html.

11. Katie Mosse, "Tom Hanks Says Type 2 Diabetes Diagnosis Spurred Weight Loss," *ABCNews*, October 8, 2013/ accessed August 3, 2014. http://abcnews.go.com/blogs/

health/2013/10/08/tom-hanks-says-type-2—diabetes-diagnosis-spurred-weight-loss/.

12. Alice Park, "Did Paula Deen's Own Cooking Give Her Diabetes"? *Time Health and Family,* January 17, 2012/accessed August 3, 2014. http://healthland.time.com/2012/01/17/did-paula-deens-own-cooking- give-her-diabetes/.

The Battle of the Bulge

1. Alan Go, Dariush Mozaffarin, Veronique Roger, Emelia Benjamin, Jarett Berry, Michael Blaha et al., "AHA Statistical Update: Heart Disease and Stroke Statistics-2014," *Circulation* 129 (2014), e89. December 18, 2014/acessed August 11, 2014. http://circ.ahajournals.org/content/early/2013/12/18/01.cir.0000441139.02102.80.

2. Rena Wing and Suzanne Phelan, "Long-term Weight Loss Maintenance," *American Journal of Clinical Nutrition* 82 (suppl) (2005): 222S-225S/accessed August 11, 2014. http://ajcn.nutrition.org/content/82/1/222S.full.pdf+html.

3. D. C. Knight, "Bowling Tips and Techniques: What Weight Bowling Ball Should You Use?," *YouTube Video*, November 1, 2009/accessed August 11, 2014.
   http://www.youtube.com/watch?v=pXvj2TiZSQg.

4. Stephen Kumanyika, Eva Obarzanek, Nicolas Stettler, Ronny Bell, Alison Field, Stephen Fortmann et al. "AHA Scientific Statement Population-Based Prevention of Obesity: The Need for Comprehensive Promotion of Healthful Eating, Physical Activity, and Energy Balance," *Circulation* 118 (2008): 428– 463/accessed August 11, 2014. http://circ.ahajournals.org/content/118/4/428.abstractDoi:10.1161/CIRCULATIONAHA.108.189702.

5. Michael Jensen, Donna Ryan, Caroline Apovian, Jamy Ard, Anthony Comuzzie, Karen Donato et al. "2013 AHA/ACC/TOS Guideline for the Management of Overweight

and Obesity in Adults: A Report of the American College of Cardiology/American Heart Association Task Force on Practice Guidelines and the Obesity Society," *Circulation*, November 12, 2013/accessed August 11, 2014. http://circ. ahajournals.org/content/early/2013/11/11/01.cir.00004377 39.71477.ee.

6. "The Practical Guide. Identification, Evaluation, and Treatment of Overweight and Obesity in Adults." *U.S. Department of Health and Human Services*, October 2000/ accessed February 5, 2015. http://www.nhlbi.gov/files/docs/ guidelines/prctgd_c.pdf

7. Brian Wansink and SeaBum Park, "At the Movies: How External Cues and Perceived Taste Impact Consumption Volume," 12, no. 1 (2000):69–74./accessed August 11, 2014. http://foodpsychology.cornell.edu/sites/default/files/ atthemovies-m 2001.pdf.

8. Brian Wansink, *Mindless Eating: Why We Eat More Than We Think* (New York, NY: Bantam Dell, 2007).

9. Brian Wansink, Koert van Ittersum and James Painter, "Ice Cream Illusions Bowls, Spoons and Self-served Portion Sizes," *American Journal of Preventive Medicine* 41, no. 3 (2006): 240–243/accessed August 11, 2014. http://mindlesseating. org/lastsupper/pdf/ice_cream_illusions_AJPM%20_2006. pdf.

10. Brian Wansink, Collin Payne and Jill North, "Fine as North Dakota Wine: Sensory Expectations and the Intake of Companion Foods," *Physiology Behavior* 90, no 5 (2007): 712–6/accessed August 11, 2014. http://foodpsychology. cornell.edu/pdf/pre-prints/ND-Wine-2007.pdf.

11. Brian Wansink, Collin Payne and Jill North, "Bottomless Bowls: Why Visual Cues of Portion Size May Influence Intake," *Obesity Research* 13, no. 1 (2005): 93– 100/accessed August 9, 2014. http://www.mindlesseating.org/lastsupper/ pdf/bottomless_soup-OR_2005.pdf.

12. Brian Wansink and Colin Payne, "Counting Bones: Environmental Cues that Decrease Food Intake," *Perceptual and Motor Skills* 104 (2007): 273–276/accessed August 9, 2014. http://www.researchgate.net/publication/6377948_Counting_bones_environmental_cues_that_decrease_food_intake.

13. Barbara Kahn and Brian Wansink, "The Influence of Assortment Structure On Perceived Variety and Consumption Quantities," *Journal of Consumer Research* 30, no. 4 (2004): 519/accessed August 9, 2014. http://mindlesseating.org/pdf/downloads/Variety-JCR_2004.pdf.

14. James Painter, Brian Wansink and Julie Hieggelke, "How Visibility and Convenience Influence Candy Consumption," *Appetite* 38, no. 3 (2002): 237–238/accessed August 11, 2014. http://foodpsychology.cornell.edu/pdf/pre-prints/candyconsumption-2002.pdf.

15. "Ebbinghaus Illusions," *New World Encyclopedia*, September 11, 2013/accessed August 11, 2014. http://www.newworldencyclopedia.org/entry/Ebbinghaus_illusion.

16. Alan Rozanski, "Integrating Psychologic Approaches into the Behavioral Management of Cardiac Patients," *Psychosomatic Medicine* 67, Supp.(2005): 1:S67– S73/accessed August 11, 2014. http://www.researchgate.net/publication/7788615_Integrating_psychologic_approaches_into_the_behavioral_management_of_cardiac_patients.

17. Oliver Grimm, "Addicited to Food? What Drives People, Against Their Better Judgment, to Eat More Food Than They Need? Scientists Look to the Brain for Answers," *Scientific American Mind* 18, (April/May 2007):36–39/ accessed August 11, 2014. http://www.nature.com/scientificamericanmind/journal/v18/n2/full/scientificameri canmind0407–36.html.

18. Anahad O'Connor, "Study Details 30–Year Increase in Calorie Consumption," *The New York Times*, February

6, 2004/accessed August 11, 2014. http://www.nytimes. com/2004/02/06/health/06CARB.html.

19. Lisa Young and Marion Nestle, "The Contribution of Expanding Portion Sizes to the US Obesity Epidemic, American Journal of Public Health, February 2002, 92 no. 2/ accessed November 23, 2014. http://www.ncbi.nlm.nih.gov/ pmc/articles/PMC1447051/pdf/0920246.pdf.

20. Preventive Cardiovascular Association (PCNA) "Portion Control," Forms/accessed August 11, 2014. http://pcna. net/clinical-tools/tools-for-healthcare-providers/download able-online-forms.

21. "USDA Choose My Plate," *United States Department of Agriculture*/accessed August 11, 2014. http://www. choosemyplate.gov/.

22. James Pochaska, John Norcross, and Carlo DiClemente, *Changing for Good: A Revolutionary Six-stage Program for Overcoming Bad Habits and Moving Your Life Positively Forward* (New York, NY: Quill, 1994), 15.

23. Kurtis Hiatt, "U.S. News and World Report Best Diets," *U.S. News and World Report*, December 12, 2013/accessed August 11, 2014. http://health.usnews.com/best-diet/ mediterranean-diet.

24. Ferris Jabr, "How to Really Eat Like a Hunter-Gatherer: Why the Paleo Diet Is Half-Baked [Interactive and Inforgraphic]," *Scientific American*, June 3, 2013/accessed August 11, 2014. http://www.scientificamerican.com/article/ why-paleo-diet-half-baked-how-hunter-gatherer-really-eat/.

25. Beth Klos, "French Paradox—Should We Be More Like the French?," *Intelihealth.com*, November 5, 2007/accessed August 11, 2014. http://www.brighamandwomens.org/Patients_ Visitors/pcs/nutrition/services/healtheweightforwomen/ special_topics/intelihealth1107.aspx?subID=submenu10.

26. Xavier Pi-Suoyu, William Dietz, Diane Becker, John Foyet, Claude Bouchard, Robert Garrison et al., "Clinical

Guidelines on the Identification, Evaluation and Treatment of Overweight and Obesity in Adults: The Evidence Report," *National Institute of Health*. September 1998. NIH 98–4083, /accessed August 11, 2014. http://www.nhlbi.nih.gov/guidelines/obesity/ob_gdlns.pdf.

27. Ferris Jabr, "Is Sugar Really Toxic? Sifting through the Evidence," *Scientific American*, July 15, 2013/accessed August 11, 2014. http://blogs.scientificamerican.com/brainwaves/2013/07/15/is-sugar-really-toxic-sifting-through-the-evidence/.

28. Cindy Fitch and Kathryn Keim, "Position of the Academy of Nutrition and Dietetics: Use of Nutritive and Nonnutritive Sweeteners," *Journal of the Academy of Nutrition and Dietetics* 112, no. 5 (2012):739–758/accessed August 11, 2015 http://www.eatright.org/About/Content.aspx?id=8363.

29. "Drinking Sugar-sweetened Beverages Daily Linked to Diabetes, Cardiovascular Disease, Increased Healthcare Costs," *American Heart Association*, March 5, 2010/acessed August 11, 2014. http://newsroom.heart.org/news/976.

30. Amanda Woerner, "The Dark Side of Diet Drinks?" *Fox News*, July 10, 2013/accessed August 11, 2014. http://www.foxnews.com/health/2013/07/10/dark-side-diet- drinks/.

31. "Low-Calorie Sweeteners," *American Diabetes Association*, January 31, 2014/accessed August 11, 2014. http://www.diabetes.org/food-and-fitness/food/what-can-i-eat/understanding-carbohydrates/artificial-sweeteners/.

32. Kelly D. Brownell, *The LEARN Program for Weight Management: Lifestyle, Exercise, Attitudes, Relationships and Nutrition*, (Dallas, TX: American Health Publishing Company, 2004).

33. Carol Porth, *Pathophysiology Concepts of Altered Health States (7th. ed.)*. (Philadelphia, PA: Lippincott Williams & Wilkins, 2005) 232.

34. George Spratto and Adrienne Woods, *Delmar Nurse's Drug Handbook*, (Clifton Park, NY: Delmar Cengage Learning, 2013).

Strategies to Help End a Tobacco Habit

1. Kathleen Sebelius, Howard Koh and Thomas Frieden, "The Health Consequences of Smoking: 50 Years of Progress A Report of the Surgeon General Executive Summary," *U.S. Department of Health and Human Services, Center for Disease Control and Prevention and Health Promotion, Office of Health*, 2014/accessed August 29, 2014. http://www.surgeongeneral. gov/library/reports/50–years-of-progress/exec-summary.pdf.

2. Linda Garrison, "Queen Mary 2 (QM2) Facts and Figures," *About Travel*, 2014/accessed August 29, 2014. http://cruises. about.com/cs/shipprofiles/a/queen_mary_5.htm.

3. "A Clinical Practice Guideline for Treating Tobacco Use and Dependence: 2008 Update," *American Journal of Preventive Medicine* 35 no. 2 (2008)/accessed November 9, 2014. http://www.ncbi.nlm.nih.gov/pubmed/18617085.

4. "Tobacco Industry," *CQ Researcher* 14 no. 43 (December 10, 2004): 1025– 1048/accessed August 29, 2014. http://www. cqpress.com/product/Researcher-Tobacco-Industry-v14–43. html.

5. Sarah Jempel, "What A Pack of Cigarettes Costs Now, State By State," *The AWL*, July 12, 2013/accessed August 29, 2014. http://www.theawl.com/2013/07/what -a-pack-of-cigarettes-costs-now-state-by-state.

6. Anita Wynne, Teri Woo and Ali Olyaei, *Pharmacotherapeutics for Nurse Practitioner Prescribers* (Philadelphia, PA: F. A. Davis Company, 2007), 174–178, 1167–1177.

7. Alan Go, Dariush Mozaffarin, Veronique Roger, Emelia Benjamin, Jarett Berry, William Borden et al., "AHA Statistical Update: Heart Disease and Stroke Statistics-2013,"

Circulation 127 (2013): e60-64/accessed August 29, 2013. http://circ.ahajournals.org/content/127/1/e6.full.pdf+html.

8. "Smoking and Tobacco Use: Bidis and Kreteks," Centers for Disease Control and Prevention, July 9, 2013/accessed November 9, 2014. http://www.cdc.gov/tobacco/data_ statistics/fact_sheets/tobacco_industry/bidis_kr eteks/.

9. "More than a Quarter-million Youth Who Had Never Smoked a Cigarette Used E-cigarettes in 2013," *CDC Centers for Disease Control and Prevention*, August 25, 2014/ accessed August 28, 2014.

10. John Heilprin, "U.N. Health Agency Urges Crackdown On E-cigarettes," *AP Yahoo News*, August 26, 2014/accessed October 11, 2014. http://news.yahoo.com/un- healthagency-e-cigarettes-must-regulated-103826438.html.

11. Abbey Race, "American Heart Association Issues E-Cigarette Recommendations," *AHA/ASA Newsroom*, August 25, 2014/ accessed August 28, 2014. http://newsroom.heart.org/ news/american-heart-association-issues-e-cigarette-recommendations?preview=4087.

12. "Who Makes Cigars: Cigar Smoking," *American Cancer Society*, January 17, 2013/accessed August 29, 2014. http:// www.cancer.org/cancer/cancercauses/tobaccocancer/ cigarsmoking/index.

13. "Smokeless Tobacco: What Is Spit or Smokeless Tobacco?," *American Cancer Society*, December 3, 2013/accessed August 29, 2014. http://www.cancer.org/cancer/cancercauses/ tobaccocancer/smokeless-tobacco.

14. A.C. Pearce and R. M. Jones, "Smoking and Anesthesia: Preoperative Abstinence and Perioperative Morbidity," *Anesthesiology* 61, no. 5 (1984): 576–584/accessed August 29, 2014. http://journals.lww.com/anesthesiology/Citation/ 1984/11000/Smoking_and_Anesthesia__Preoperative_ Abstinence.18.aspx.

15. Cindy Tumiel, "Clot Study Shows Cigarette Could Trigger Heart Attack," March 18, 2001, *Chicago Tribune*/accessed August 29, 2014. http://articles.chicagotribune.com/2001–03–18/news/0103180438_1_blood-clots- factors-for-heart-disease-coronary-artery.

16. "Surgeon General Report: Section Three Secondhand Smoke," *A Guide for Counseling Women Who Smoke*, Winter 2008/accessed August 29, 2014. http://whb.ncpublichealth.com/Manuals/counseling/Secondhand-Smoke.pdf.

17. "Secondhand Smoke (SHS) Facts," *Center for Disease Control and Prevention*, March 4, 2014/accessed August 29, 2014. http://www.cdc.gov/tobacco/data_statistics/fact_sheets/secondhand_smoke/general_facts.

18. "Addictions," *American Psychological Association*, 2014/accessed April 1, 2014. http://www.apa.org/topics/addiction/.

19. James Wright, "The Health Consequences of Smoking: Nicotine Addiction: The Report of the Surgeon General (1988)," *U.S. Department of Health and Human Services*, (1988)/accessed August 29, 2014. http://profiles.nlm.nih.gov/NN/B/B/Z/D/.

20. Michael Fiore, Carlos Jaen, Timothy Bake, William Bailey, Neal Benowitz, Susan Curry et al., "Quick Reference Guide for Clinicians 2008 Update: Treating Tobacco Use and Dependence," *U.S. Department of Health and Human Services, Public Health Services* (April 2009)/accessed August 29, 2014. http://www.uclahealth.org/workfiles/smoke-free/treating-tobacco-dependenc.pdf.

21. George Spratto and Adrienne Woods, *Delmar Nurse's Drug Handbook*, (Clifton Park, NY: Delmar Cengage Learning, 2013).

22. "Smokeless Tobacco: A Guide for Quitting," *National Institute of Health (NIH) Publication*, August 2012/accessed August 29, 2014. http://www.nidcr.nih.gov/oralhealth/Topics/

SmokelessTobacco/SmokelessTobacc oAGuideforQuitting. htm.

Physical Activity: Use It or Lose It

1. Alan Go, Dariush Mozaffarin, Veronique Roger, Emelia Benjamin, Jarett Berry, Michael Blaha et al., "AHA Statistical Update: Heart Disease and Stroke Statistics-2014," *Circulation* 129 (2014): e65, December 18, 2014/accessed May 19, 2014. http://circ.ahajournals.org/content/early/2013/12/18/01.cir. 0000441139.02102.80.

2. Bruno Balke and James Peterson, *The Stairmaster Fitness Handbook, (2nd. ed).* (Champaign, IL: Sagamore Publishing, Inc., 1995), 57.

3. "PAR-Q-The Physical Activity Readiness Questionnaire," *Canadian Society for Exercise Physiology*, 2014/accessed September 9, 2014. http://www.csep.ca/english/view.asp? x=698.

4. Robert Eckel, John Jakicic, Jamy Ard, Van Hubbard, Janet de Jesus, I-Min Lee, Alice Lichtenstein et al., "2013 AHA/ ACC Guidelines on Lifestyle Management to Reduce Cardiovascular Risk: A Report of the American College of Cardiology/American Heart Association Task Force on Practice Guidelines," *Circulation*, November 12, 2013/ accessed September 9, 2014, http://circ.ahajournals.org/ content/early/2013/11/11/01.cir.0000437740.48606.d1.

5. Lawrence Armstrong, Gary Balady, Michael Berry, Shala Davis, Brenda Davy, Kevin Davy, Barry Franklin et al., *American College of Sport's Medicine's (ACSM) Guidelines for Exercise Testing and Prescription (7th ed).* (Baltiomre MD: Lippincott Williams and Wilkins, 2006, 141 and 303).

6. "Target Heart Rates," *American Heart Association*, March 22, 2013/accessed October 11, 2014. http://www.heart. org/HEARTORG/GettingHealthy/PhysicalActivity/

FitnessBasics/Target-Heart-Rates_UCM_434341_Article.
jsp.

7. "Physical Activity: Measuring Physical Activity Intensity,"
    CDC Centers for Disease Control and Prevention, December
    1, 2011/accessed September 9, 2014. http://www.cdc.gov/
    physicalactivity/everyone/measuring/.

8. "Lifestyle Interventions: Physical Activity," *National
    Guidelines and Tools for Cardiovascular Risk Reduction: A Pocket
    Guide*, Preventive Cardiovascular Nurses Association (Irving
    Place, NY: Philips Healthcare Communications, 2009). (46)

9. "Warning Signs of a Heart Attack," *American Heart
    Association*, 2012/accessed November 8, 2013. http://
    www.heart.org/HEARTORG/Conditions/HeartAttack/
    WarningSignso faHeartAttack/Warning-Signs-of-a-Heart-
    Attack_UCM_002039_Article.jsp.

10. "Stroke Warning Signs and Symptoms," *American Stroke
    Association*, 2013/accessed November 8, 2013. http://
    strokeassociation.org/STROKEORG/WarningSigns/
    Stroke-Warning-Signs-percent09and-Symptoms_
    UCM_308528_SubHomePage.jsp.

11. "What Is the Heat Index?," *National Weather Service Weather
    Forecast Office*, February 26, 2014/accessed September 9,
    2014. http://www.srh.noaa.gov/ama/?n=heatindex.

12. Charles Carpenter, Robert Griggs and Joseph Loscalzo,
    "*CECIL Essentials of Medicine (6th ed)*. (Philadelphia, PA: W.
    B. Saunders, 2004, 822 and 1106).

13. "Heat Related Deaths-Chicago, Illinois, 1996–2001, and
    United States, 1979–1999," *CDC: MMWR Weekly*, July 4,
    2003/accessed September 9, 2014. http://www.cdc.gov/
    mmwr/preview/mmwrhtml/mm5226a2.htm.

14. "Evidence Growing of Air Pollution's Link To Heart Disease,
    Death," *American Heart Association Scientific Statement*, May
    10, 2010/accessed September 9, 2014. http://newsroom.
    heart.org/news/1029.

15. "Air Quality Index (AQI)- A Guide To Air Quality and Your Health," *Air Now*, April 1, 2014/accesed September 9, 2014. http://airnow.gov/index.cfm?action=aqibasics.aqi.

16. "Physical Activity In Older Americans," *American Heart Association*, April 30, 2014/accessed September 9, 2014. http://www.heart.org/HEARTORG/GettingHealthy/PhysicalActivity/Getting Active/Exercise-Tips-for-Older-Americans_UCM_308039_Article.jsp.

17. Edward Archer, Robin Shook, Diana Thomas, Timothy Church, Peter Katzmarzk, James Hebert et al., "45–Year Trends In Women's Use of Time and Household Management Energy Expenditure," *PLOS ONE* 8 no. 2 (2013)/accessed September 9, 2014. http://www.plosone.org/article/info%3Adoi%2F10.1371%2Fjournal.pone.005662 0.

18. Jason Andrade and Andrew Ignaszewski, "Exercise and the Heart: A Review of the Early Studies, in Memory of Dr. R. S. Paffenbarger," *British Columbia Medical Journal* 49 no. 10 (2007), accessed September 9, 2014. http://ww.bcmj.org/article/exercise-and-heart-review-early-studies-memory-dr-m rs-paffenbarger.

19. "2008 Physical Activity Guidelines for Americans," *U. S. Department Health and Human Services*, ODPHP Publication No. U0036, October 2008/accessed September 9, 2014. http://www.health.gov/paguidelines/pdf/paguide.pdf.

20. David Eagleman, *Incognito: The Secret Lives of the Brain* (New York: NY: Random House, 2011).

21. Lorie Johnson, "Get Off Your Duff! Sitting Is the New Smoking," *CBN News*, November 28, 2012/Accessed July 5, 2014. http://www.cbn.com/cbnnews/healthscience/2012/june/get-off-your-duff-sitting- the-new-smoking/.

Controlling Your Response to Life's Stressors

1. Alan Rozanski, James Blumenthal, Katina Davidson, Patrice Saab and Laura Kubzansky, "State of the Art Paper: The Epidemiology, Pathophysiology, and Management of Psychosocial Risk Factors in Cardiac Practice, The Emerging Field of Behavioral Cardiology," *Journal of the American College of Cardiology* 45 no. 5 (2005): 637–651/accessed August 31, 2014. http://content.onlinejacc.org/article.aspx?articleid=1136408.

2. David Goldstein, "Walter Cannon: Homeostasis, the Fight-or-Flight Response, the Sympathoadrenal System, and the Wisdom of the Body," *Brain Immune and Resource Bridging and Immunology*, May 16, 2009/accessed August 31, 2014. http://brainimmune.com/walter-cannon-homeostasis-the-fight-or-flight-response- the-sympathoadrenal-system-and-the-wisdom-of-the-body/.

3. Hans Selye, "Stress and the General Adaptation Syndrome," *British Medical Journal*, June 17, 1950/accessed August 31, 2014. http://www.ncbi.nlm.nih.gov/pmc/articles/PMC2038 162/pdf/brmedj03603– 0003.pdf.

4. Linda Witek-Janusek, Kevin Albuquerque, Karen Chronial, Christopher Chroniak, Ramon Durazo and Herbert Matthews, "Effect of Mindfulness Based Stress Reduction on Immune Function, Quality of Life and Coping in Women Newly Diagnosed with Early Stage Breast Cancer," *Brain Behavior Immunology* 22, no. 6 (2008): 969–981/accessed August 31, 2014 http://www.ncbi.nlm.nih.gov/pmc/articles/PMC2586059/.

5. Janice Kiecolt-Glaser, Lyanne McGuire, Theodore Robles and Ronald Glaser, "Emotions, Morbidity, and Mortality: New Perspectives in Psychoneuroimmunolgy," *Annual Review of Psychology* 53,(2002): 83– 107/accessed August

31, 2014. http://www.annualreviews.org/doi/abs/10.1146/annurev.psych.53.100901.135217.

6. Meryl Hyman Harris, "Hard Marriages Can Harden Arteries," *Health Day News for Healthier Living*," March 3, 2006/accessed August 31, 2014. http://consumer.healthday.com/circulatory-system-information-7/coronary-and-artery-news-356/hard-marriages-can-harden-arteries-531357.html.

7. Lindsey Tanner, "Study Ties Marital Strife, Heart Disease," *USA Today*, October 9, 2007/accessed August 31, 2014. http://usatoday30.usatoday.com/news/health/2007–10–08–2406893824_x.htm.

8. Todd Neale, "Heart Attacks Up in Katrina's Aftermath," *Medpage Today*, August 31, 2014/accessed May 26, 2014. http://www.medpagetoday.com/Cardiology/Myocardial Infarction/44903.

9. Gene Emery, "Cardiac Arrests Peaked after Record Japanese Earthquake," *Reuters*, November 27, 2013/accessed August 31, 2014. http://www.reuters.com/article/2013/11/27/us-car diac-arrests- idUSBRE9AQ1B520131127.

10. Jonathan Steinberg, Aysha Arshad, Marcin Kowalski, Valentin Suma, Margot Vloka et al., "Increased Incidence of Life-Threatening Ventricular Arrhythmias in Implantable Defibrillator Patients after the World Trade Center Attack," *Electrophysiology* 44 no. 6 (2004): 1261–1264/accessed August 31, 2014. http://content.onlinejacc.org/article.aspx?articleid=1135955.

11. "5 Simple Heart Healthy Energy Boosters," *American Heart Association*, March 9, 2014/accessed August 31, 2014. http://www.heart.org/HEARTORG/GettingHealthy/5–Simple-Heart-Healthy-Energy-Boosters_UCM_434961_Article.jsp.

12. E. Sharman, J. R. Cockroft and J. S. Coombes, "Cardiovascular Implications of Exposure to Traffic Air Pollution During

Exercise," *Quarterly Journal of Medicine* 97, no. 10 (2004), Accessed May 19, 2014. http://www.ncbi.nlm.nih.gov/pub med/15367733.

13. L Sher, "Type D Personality: The Heart, Stress, and Cortisol," *Quarterly Journal of Medicine* 98 (2005): 323–329/ accessed August 31, 2014. http://www.uic.edu/classes/psych/ Health/Readings/Sher,%20Type%20D%20overveiw,%20 QJMed,%202005.pdf.

14. Nina Kupper and Johan Denollet, "Type D Personality as a Prognostic Factor In Heart Disease: Assessment and Mediating Mechanisms," *Journal of Personality Assessment* 89, no. 3 (2007): 265–276/accessed August 31, 2014. http:// www.ncbi.nlm.nih.gov/pubmed/18001227.

15. Yoichi Chida and Andrew Steptoe, "The Association of Anger and Hostility with Future Coronary Heart Disease," *Journal of the American College of Cardiology* 53, no. 11 (2009): 936– 946/accessed August 31, 2014. http://content.onlinejacc.org/ article.aspx?articleid=1139524.

16. Wolfgang Linden, Melanie Phillips and Jocelyne Leclerc, "Psychological Treatment of Cardiac Patients: A Meta-analysis," *European Heart Journal* 28 (2007): 2972– 2984/ accessed August 31, 2014. http://www.ncbi.nlm.nih.gov/ pubmedhealth/PMH0025222/.

Overcoming Barriers to Change

1. Jonathan Goldman, *Webster's New World Pocket Dictionary (4th ed)*. (United States: Wiley Publishing, Inc. 2000), 269.

2. James Pochaska, John Norcross, and Carlo DiClemente, *Changing for Good: A Revolutionary Six-stage Program for Overcoming Bad Habits and Moving Your Life Positively Forward* (New York, NY: Quill, 1994), 15.

3. Stephen Rollnick, Pip Mason and Chris Butler, *Health Behavior Change, A Guide for Practitioners* (China: Churchill Livingston, 1999), 73.

4. Heather Lett, James Blumenthal, Michael Babyak, Timothy Strauman, Clive Robins and Andrew Less, "Social Support and Coronary Heart Disease: Epidemiologic Evidence and Implications for Treatment," *Psychosomatic Medicine* 67, no. 6 (2005) 869–878/accessed September 2, 2014. http://www.ncbi.nlm.nih.gov/pubmed/16314591.

5. Alan Rozanski, "Integrating Psychologic Approaches into the Behavioral Management of Cardiac Patients," *Psychosomatic Medicine* 67, supplement 1 (2005): S67–S73/accessed August 31, 2014. http://journals.lww.com/psychosomaticmedicine/Abstract/2005/05001/Integrating_Psychologic_Approaches_Into_the.16.aspx.

6. Carol Ferrans, "Development of a Quality of Life Index for Patients with Cancer," *Oncology Nursing Forum* 17 no. 3 (1990): 15–19/accessed September 2, 2014. http://www.ncbi.nlm.nih.gov/pubmed/2342979.

7. Jennie Johnson, *Risk Perception, Psychological Well-being and Health-promoting Behaviors in Persons Informed of a Coronary Artery Calcium Score* (Ann Arbor, MI, 2012)/accessed September 2, 2014. http://ecommons.luc.edu/luc_diss/304/.

8. "Shop Jazzercize," *Jazzercize*/accessed September 2, 2014. http://www.jazzercize.com/shop/home-workout-dvds.

9. Denise Mann, "Cash Incentives, Penalties, May Spur People to Shed More Pounds," *Health Day*, March 7, 2013/accessed September 2, 2014. http://consumer.healthday.com/mental-health-information-25/behavior-health- news-56/cash-incentives-penalties-may-spur-people-to-shed-more-pounds- 674193.html.

10. Bill Hendrick, "WebMD Financial Incentives Help Smokers Quit," *CardioSmart, American College of Cardiology*, February 11, 2009/accessed September 2, 2014. http://

www.webmd.com/smoking-cessation/news/20090210/ financial- incentives-help-smokers-quit.

11. "A Word About Success Rates for Quitting Smoking," *American Cancer Society*, February 6, 2014/accessed September 2, 2014. http://www.cancer.org/healthy/stayaway fromtobacco/guidetoquittingsmoking/guide-to-quitting -smoking-success-rates.

12. Kathleen Sebelius, Howard Koh and Thomas Frieden, "The Health Consequences of Smoking: 50 Years of Progress A Report of the Surgeon General Executive Summary," *U.S. Department of Health and Human Services, Center for Disease Control and Prevention and Health Promotion, Office of Health*, 2014/accessed August 29, 2014. http://www.surgeongeneral. gov/library/reports/50–years-of-progress/exec-summary.pdf.

13. Eva Lonn, Jackie Bosch, Koon Teo, Prem Pais, Dennis Xavier and Salim Yusuf, "The Polypill in the Prevention of Cardiovascular Disease: Key Concepts, Current Status, Challenges and Future Directions," *Circulation* 122 (2010) 2078–2088/accessed September 2, 2014. http://circ.aha journals.org/content/122/20/2078.full.pdf+html.

14. Susan Bastable, *Nurse as Educator: Principles of Teaching and Learning for Nursing Practice*, (Jones and Bartlett Publishers, Sudbury, MA, 2003) 542.

Working With Your Healthcare Provider

1. "Medical Assistant Training-What You Can Expect," *Medical Assistant Career*/accessed September 10, 2014. http://www. medical-assistant- career.com/training/.

2. "What Is A Licensed Practical Nurse (LPN)?" *Licensed Practical Nurse*, (2014)/accessed September 10, 2014. http:// www.licensedpracticalnurse.net/what-is-an-lpn/.

3. "The Registered Nurse Population: Initial Findings from the Initiation on the Future of Nursing," *U. S. Department*

of Health and Human Services (13), March 2010/accessed November 7, 2014. http://www.thefutureofnursing.org/resource/detail/registered-nurse-population-findings-2008-national-sample-survey-registered-nurses.

4. "Fact Sheet: The Doctor of Nursing Practice," *American Association of Colleges of Nursing*, August 18, 2014/accessed September 10, 2014. http://www.aacn.nche.edu/media-relations/fact-sheets/dnp.

5. "Hiring A Physician Assistant or Nurse Practitioner," *Center for Practice Improvement and Innovation, American College of Physicians*, February 2010/accessed September 10, 2014. http://www.acponline.org/running_practice/practice_management/human_resources/panp2.pdf.

6. "Requirements for Becoming A Physician,"*American Medical Association*/accessed September 10, 2014. http://www.ama-assn.org/ama/pub/education-careers/becoming-physician.page?

7. Peter Lockhart, Ann Bolger, Panos Papapanou, Olusegun Osinbowale, Maurizio Trevisan, Matthew Levison et al., "Periodontal Disease and Atherosclerotic Vascular Disease: Does the Evidence Support an Independent Association?: A Scientific Statement from the American Heart Association," *Circulation* 125 (2012): 2520–2544/accessed September 10, 2014. http://circ.ahajournals.org/content/125/20/2520.full.pdf+html.

8. Vincent Friedwald, Kenneth Kornman, James Beck, Robert Genco, Allison Goldfine, Peter Libby et al., "The American Journal of Cardiology and Journal of Periodontal Editors' Consensus: Periodontitis and Atherosclerotic Cardiovascular Disease," *American Journal of Cardiology* 105 (2009):59–68/accessed September 10, 2014 http://www.eauclaireperiodontics.com/pdfs/cardio_paper.17123103.pdf.

9. Sidney Smith, Emelia Benjamin, Robert Bonow, Lynne Braun, Mark Creager, Barry Franklin, Raymond Gibbons

et al., "AHA/ACC Secondary Prevention and Risk Reduction Therapy for Patients with Coronary and Other Atherosclerotic Vascular Disease: 2011 Update: A Guideline from the American Heart Association and American College of Cardiology Foundation," *Circulation*, 124 (2011): 2458–2473. http://circ.ahajournals.org/content/124/22/2458.full. pdf+html.

Research and Websites You Can Trust

1. Marcia Stanhope and Jeanette Lancaster, *Foundations of Nursing in the Community Oriented Practice* (St. Louis, MO: Mosby Elsevier, 2006), 158.
2. S.P. Stone, "Hand Hygiene-the Case for Evidenced-based Education," *Journal of the Royal Society of Medicine*, 94, (2001): 278–281/accessed August 21, 2014. http://www.ncbi.nlm. nih.gov/pmc/articles/PMC1281522/pdf/0940278.pdf.
3. *"Nursing's Social Policy Statement (2nd ed.)* (Silver Spring, MD, 2003), 35.
4. Agnes Ullman, "Louis Pastuer," *Encyclopedia Britannica*, June 6, 2014/accessed August 23, 2014. http://www.britannica. com/EBchecked/topic/445964/Louis-Pasteur.
5. "A Century Gone-Sir Joseph Lister, Bt. (1827–1912): Antisepsis and the Beginnings of Modern Surgical Medicine," *Museum of Health Care Blog*, February 10, 2012/accessed August 23, 2014. http://museumofhealthcare.wordpress. com/2012/02/10/sir-joseph-lister/.
6. "John Snow (1813–1858)," *BBC History*/accessed August 23, 2014. http://www.bbc.co.uk/history/historic_figures/snow_ john.shtml.
7. Nancy Burns and Susan Grove, *The Practice of Nursing Research: Appraisal, Synthesis, and Generation of Evidence (6th ed.)* (St. Louis, MO: Saunders Elsevier, 2005), 207, 357.

8. "Paleo Diet," *U.S. News and World Report, Health and Wellness*/accessed August 23, 2014. http://health.usnews.com /best-diet/paleo-diet.

9. Robb Wolf, "The Paleo Diet-Robb Wolf On Paleolithic Nutrition, *Intermittent Fasting, and Fitness*," June 11, 2011/ accessed August 23, 2014. http://robbwolf.com/2011/06/11/ us-news-best-diets-rebuttal-2/.

10. Nina Teicholz, "The Questionable Link Between Saturated Fat and Heart Disease," *The Wall Street Journal*, May 6, 2014/ accessed August 23, 2014. http://online.wsj.com/news/articles/ SB10001424052702303677840457953 3760760481486.

11. Alan Go, Dariush Mozaffarin, Veronique Roger, Emelia Benjamin, Jarett Berry, Michael Blaha et al., "AHA Statistical Update: Heart Disease and Stroke Statistics-2014," *Circulation* 129 (2014): December 18, 2014/acessed August 23, 2014. http://circ.ahajournals.org/content/early/2013/12/18/01.cir. 0000441139.02102.80.

12. Rajiv Chowdhury, Samantha Warnakula, Setor Kunutsor, Francesca Crowe, Heather Ward, Laura Johnson et al., "Association of Dietary, Circulating, and Supplement Fatty Acids with Coronary Risk: A Systematic Review and Meta-analysis," *University of York Centre for Reviews and Dissemination*/accessed August 23, 2014. http://annals.org/ article.aspx?articleid=1846638.

13. Jacque Rossouw, Garnet Anderson, Ross Prentice, Andrea LaCroix, Charles Kooperberg, Marcia Stefanick et al., "Risks and Benefits of Estrogen Plus Progestin in Healthy Postmenopausal Women: Principal Result from the Women's Health Initiative Randomize Controlled Trial," *Journal of the American Medical Association* 288, no. 3 (2002), accessed August 23, 2014.http://jama.jamanetwork.com/article.aspx? articleid=195120.

14. Marina Johnson, *Outliving Your Ovaries: An Endocrinologist Weighs the Risks and Rewards of Treating Menopause with*

Hormone Replacement Therapy (Irving, Texas: Eyesong Publishing, 2011, 96, 129, 134).

15. "About the American Heart Association: Our Mission," *American Heart Association*/accessed August 23, 2014. http://www.heart.org/HEARTORG/General/About-Us—American-Heart-m Association_UCM_305422_SubHome Page.jsp.

16. Claude Lenfant and Jay Moskowitz, "The National Heart, Lung and Blood Institute: A Plan for the Eighties," *Circulation* 68 (1983): 1141/accessed June 21, 2014. http://circ.ahajournals.org/content/68/5/1141.full.pdf.

17. "NHLBI Mission Statement," *National, Heart, Lung and Blood Institute*, June 2009/accessed August 23, 2014. http://www.nhlbi.nih.gov/about/org/mission.htm.

A Word to Healthcare Providers

1. Alan Go, Dariush Mozaffarin, Veronique Roger, Emelia Benjamin, Jarett Berry, Michael Blaha et al., "AHA Statistical Update: Heart Disease and Stroke Statistics-2014," *Circulation* 129 (2014), e217, December 18, 2014/accessed August 11, 2014. http://circ.ahajournals.org/content/early/2013/12/18/01.cir.0000441139.02102.80.

2. "Rescuing A Besieged City: A Closer Look At Patient Self-care Challenges," *Cardiology*, *Spring 2013*/accessed August 21, 2014. http://www.cardiosource.org/~/media/Files/News%20and%20Media/Car dioSource%20and%20 Cardiology%20News%20Media/2013/05/Cardiomag _Sp13 _SELF-CARE2.

3. Stephen Rollnick, William Miller and Christopher Butler, *Motivational Interviewing in Health Care*, (New York, NY: Guilford Publications, 2008).

4. B. Plassman, K. Langa, G. Fisher, S. Heeringa, D. Weir, M. Ofstedal et al., "Prevalence of Dementia In the United

States: The Aging, Demographics, and Memory Study," *Neuroepidemiology* 29 (2007): 125–132/accessed August 21, 2014. http://www.ncbi.nlm.nih.gov/pubmed/17975326.

5. Judith Lichtman, Thomas Bigger, James Blumenthal, Nancy Frasure-Smith, Peter Kaufmann, Francois Lesperance et al., "Depression and Coronary Heart Disease: Recommendations for Screening, Referral, and Treatment: A Science Advisory from the American Heart Association Prevention Committee of the Council on Cardiovascular Nursing, Council on Clinical Cardiology, Council on Epidemiology and Prevention, and Interdisciplinary Council on Quality of Care and Outcomes Research: Endorsed by the American Psychiatric Association," *Circulation* 118 (2008): 1768–1775/accessed August 21, 2014. http://circ.ahajournals.org/content/118/17/1768.full.pdf+html.

6. Alan Rozanski, "Integrating Psychologic Approaches into the Behavioral Management of Cardiac Patients," *Psychosomatic Medicine* 67, supplement 1 (2005): S67– S73/accessed August 21, 2014. http://www.researchgate.net/publication/7788615_Integrating_psychologic _approaches_into_the_behavioral_management_of_cardiac_patients.

7. Leslie Moore, Laura Kimble, and Ptlene Minick, "Perceptions of Cardiac Risk Factors and Risk-reduction Behavior in Women with Known Coronary Heart Disease," *Journal of Cardiovascular Nursing* 25 no. 6 (2010): 433–443/accessed August 21, 2014. http://www.ncbi.nlm.nih.gov/pubmed/20938247.

8. Lawrence Phillips, William Branch, Curtiss Cook, Joyce Doyle, Imad El-Kebbi, Daniel Gallina et al., "Clinical Inertia," *Annals of Internal Medicine* 135, no 9 (2001)/accessed August 21, 2014. http://annals.org/article.aspx?articleid=714878.

9. "Physician Behavior and Practice Patterns Related To Smoking Cessation. Full Report," *Association of American Medical Colleges*, 2007/accessed August 21, 2014. http://

www.legacyforhealth.org/content/download/566/6812/file/
Physicians_Stud y.pdf.

10. Mary Waring, Mary Roberts, Donna Parker and Charles
Eaton, "Documentation and Management of Overweight
and Obesity in Primary Care," *Journal of the American Board
of Family Medicine* 22, no. 5 (2009): 547/accessed August
21, 2014. http://www.jabfm.org/content/22/5/544.full.pdf+
html.

11. James Pochaska, John Norcross, and Carlo DiClemente,
*Changing for Good: A Revolutionary Six-stage Program for
Overcoming Bad Habits and Moving Your Life Positively
Forward* (New York, NY: Quill, 1994), 15.

12. Michael Jensen, Donna Ryan, Caroline Apovian, Jamy Ard,
Anthony Comuzzie, Karen Donato et al. "2013 AHA/
ACC/TOS Guideline for the Management of Overweight
and Obesity in Adults: A Report of the American College
of Cardiology/American Heart Association Task Force on
Practice Guidelines and the Obesity Society," *Circulation*,
November 12, 2013/accessed August 21, 2014. http://circ.
ahajournals.org/content/early/2013/11/11/01.cir.00004377
39. 71477.ee.

13. Michael Fiore, Carlos Jaen, Timothy Bake, William Bailey,
Neal Benowitz, Susan Curry et al., "Quick Reference Guide
for Clinicians 2008 Update: Treating Tobacco Use and
Dependence," *U.S. Department of Health and Human Services,
Public Health Services* (April 2009)/accessed August 21, 2014.
http://www.uclahealth.org/workfiles/smoke-free/treating-
tobacco- dependence.pdf.

14. Rita Redberg, Emelia Benjamin, Vera Bittner, Lynne Braun,
David Goff, and Stephen Havas, S. et al. "ACCF/AHA
2009 Performance Measures for Primary Prevention of
Cardiovascular Disease in Adults," *Journal of the American
College of Cardiology* 120(2009): 1296–1336/accessed August
21, 2014. http://circ.ahajournals.org/content/120/13/1296.full.

15. Ira Ockene, Laura Hayman, Richard Pasternak, Eleanor Schron and Jacqueline Dunbar-Jacob, "Task Force #4 Adherence Issues and Behavior Changes: Achieving A Long-term Solution," *Journal of the American College of Cardiology* 40 no. 4 (2002): 630–640/accessed August 21, 2014. http://content.onlinejacc.org/article.aspx?articleid=1130308.

16. Elizabeth Stewart and Chester Fox, "Encouraging Patients to Change Unhealthy Behaviors with Motivational Interviewing," *Family Practice Management*," 18 no. 3 (May/June 2011):21–25/accessed August 21, 2014. http://www.aafp.org/fpm/2011/0500/p21.html.

17. Suzanne Arnold, John Spertus, Frederick Masoudi, Stacie Daughtery, Thomas Maddox, John Dodson et al., "Beyond Medication Prescription As Performance Measures: Optimal Secondary Prevention Medication Dosing after Acute Myocardial Infarction," *Journal of the American College of Cardiology*, 62 no. 19 (2013): 1791–1801/accessed August 21, 2014. http://content.onlinejacc.org/article.aspx?articleid=1731143.

18. Sidney Smith, Emelia Benjamin, Robert Bonow, Lynne Braun, Mark Creager, Barry Franklin et al., "AHA/ACCF Secondary Prevention and Risk Reduction Therapy for Patients with Coronary and Atherosclerotic Vascular Disease: 2011 Update: A Guideline from the American Heart Association and the American College of Cardiology," *Circulation* 124 November 3, 2011:2458–2473/ accessed August 21, 2014. http://circ.ahajournals.org/content/124/22/2458.full.pdf+html.

19. "The Mission of the Preventive Cardiovascular Nurses Association,"/accessed June 29, 2014. http://pcna.net/about/our-mission.

20. Jennie Johnson, *Risk Perception, Psychological Well-being and Health-promoting Behaviors in Persons Informed of a Coronary Artery Calcium Score* (Ann Arbor, MI, 2012)/accessed August 21, 2014. http://ecommons.luc.edu/luc_diss/304/.

21. Philip Greenland, Robert Bonow, Bruce Brundage, Matthew Budoff, Mark Eisenberg et al., "ACC/AHA 2007 Clinical Expert Consensus Document on Coronary Artery Calcium Scoring by Computed Tomography in Global Cardiovascular Risk Assessment and in Evaluation of Patients with Chest Pain," *Circulation* 115 (2007): 402–426.

Closing Thoughts (no references)

Index

A

5 As, 300
ACE inhibitors, 97
Addiction quiz, 188; 195
Aerobic exercise, 201–202; 207–211
Agaidika Shoshone tribal woman, 285
Aging, 219–220
Air pollution, 219
Alcohol, 96; 164
Altitude, 217–219
Ambivalence, 244–245; 294; 298–299
American Heart Association, 282
Anger, 237–239
Angiogram/catheterization, 25
Angiotensin receptor blockers, 97–98
Artificial sweeteners, 162–163
Asymptomatic disease, 289–291
Atkins diet, 155

B

Bariatric surgery, 165
Barriers, 241–259
Beta-blocker, 98
Berry, Halley, 121–122
Bidis, 176
Binge eating, 145–146
Blood pressure, 79–101
    -Machine, 87
    -Technique, 88–89
Blood test
    -C reactive protein, 49–50
    -Cholesterol, 57
    -Cotinine, 181–182
    -Hemoglobin A1C, 115
    -Sugar, 114
Body mass index (BMI), 127–129; 325–327
Boredom, 137–138; 249
Bottomless Soup Bowl Study, 133
Bush, George, 51–52
Bupropion/Zyban, 191–192

C

Caffeine, 94–96
Caffeine powder, 95
Calcium channel blockers, 98
Calcium deposits, 34–35
Calories, 142; 153; 158; 211
Cardiac rehabilitation, 25–26
Carnegie, Dale, 19
Catheterization of heart, 25
Certified medical assistant, 262
Changing, 246; 295

Chantix, 192–194

Chocolate cake serving, 153

Cholesterol numbers, 55–61

Choose My Plate, 140–142

Cigarette chemicals, 173–174

Cigars, 177–178

Clark, Dave, 52

Clinical inertia, 292

Cognitive impairments, 255-256

Cold wind chill index, 217; 331

Comfort foods men/women, 135–136

Communication techniques, 266–267

Confidence ruler, 246; 294

Cooldowns, 206–207

Coop, Everett, 79

Coping with stressors, 233–237

Coronary artery bypass graft surgery, 25

Coronary artery calcium heart scan, 45–49

Cost barriers, 256–257

C Reactive Protein, 49–50

CPR, 26–27

Coronary arteries, 21–22

Cravings, 143–146, 184, 187–188, 248

Cuff size, 87–88

Cutler, Jay, 120–121

D

Daily weights, 151

DASH diet, 93–94; 157–158

Deen, Paula, 122–123

Denial, 39–40; 243–244; 293–294

Dental hygiene, 268–270

Deep breathing technique, 234

Depression, 137-138, 250-251, 288-289
Dessert, 149–151
Diabetes, 103–124
      -Type 1, 105–107
      -Type 2, 108–111
Diabetes Prevention Trial, 115–116
Doctor/physician, 266
Dot test, 136–137

E

E-cigarettes, 176–177
End organ damage (high BP), 84
Energy production, 200–201
Environmental barriers, 253–254
Eye damage (diabetes), 111
Exercise, 152; 199–226

F

Family eating (healthier), 159-160
Farmer story, 53
Fasting blood sugar, 114
Financial barriers, 252–253
Fixx, James, 50–51
Food label
      -Butter, 66–68
      -Ice cream, 64; 139
      -Milk, 65–66
      -Portion control, 138–142
      -Potato chips, 92
      -Trans-fats, 66–68
      -Salt/sodium, 90–93
      -Saturated fat, 62–66

Ford, Henry, 241
Framingham Heart Study, 40–41
Fruits and vegetables, 93–94
Fuller, Thomas, 306

G

Gandolfini, James, 51
Gestational diabetes, 110–111
Glucose tolerance test (oral), 114–115

Gum (nicotine), 190

H

Habit, 224–225
Halo Effect, 152–153
Hanks, Tom, 122
Hardening of the arteries, 31–35
HDL cholesterol, 58–59
Healthcare providers, 261–270, 285–306
Healthy Eating
        -Cholesterol, 61–71
        -Families, 159–160
        -Holidays, 151
        -Salt, 89–93
        -Weight, 125–167
Heart attack, 19–36
Heart disease
        -Anatomy/physiology, 19–22
        -Catheterization/angiogram, 25
Heart Attack Risk Calculator, 44; 73–74
Heat exhaustion/heat stroke, 215–217
Heat index, 215; 330

Hemoglobin A1C, 115
Hershey Kisses Temptation Study, 134–135
High blood pressure/hypertension, 79–101
       -Damage, 83–84
       -Emergencies, 83
       -Measurement, 85–89
       -Pregnancy induced, 85
       -Primary HTN, 84–85
       -Secondary HTN, 85
High blood sugar, 117–118
High fructose corn syrup, 161–162
Holidays, 151; 237
Home BP monitoring, 85–89
Hormone replacement therapy, 279–282
Hostility, 237–239
Hypoglycemia/hyperglycemia, 117–118

I

Ice Cream Social study, 132
Illiteracy, 256, 286–287
Illusion of size, 136–137
Imagery, 235
Inflammation test, 49–50
Influenza, 270
Inhaler (nicotine), 190–191
Institutional review board, 274–275
Insulin, 105; 116–118
Insulin Resistance, 108–109
Intensity of exercise, 204–211

J

Jennie's top 10 list (weight control), 166
Jenny Craig, 156
Johnson, Jennie research study, 303–305
Johnson, Marina, 280–282
Julie Cake recipe, 150

K

Kidney damage (diabetes), 112

L

LDL cholesterol, 31–35; 56–76
Letterman, David, 51
Licensed practical nurse, 262–263
Liquid food, 147
Lister, Joseph, 273
Living for a Healthy Heart Plan, 69–71; 158–159
Lovecraft, H. P., 37
Low blood sugar, 117
Lozenge (nicotine), 190

M

Maintaining change, 247; 295–296
Media barriers, 253
Medications
        -Adherence, 255–258; 301–302
        -Blood pressure, 97–101
        -Cholesterol, 71–76
        -Diabetes, 105–109; 116–118
        -Smoking, 189–194

Mediterranean diet, 156–157
Metabolic syndrome, 119
Milk example, 65–66
M and M Color Temptation study, 134
Monounsaturated fats (oils), 69
Moore, Mary Tyler, 120
Motivational interviewing, 296–300
My Food Pyramid, 140–142

N

National, Heart, Lung, and Blood Institute, 282
Negative mood, 137–138
Nerve damage (diabetes), 112
Nicotine
       -Addiction, 184–188; 195–196
       -Blood levels, 188
       -Spray, 191
       -Replacements, 189–191
Niebuhr, Reinhold, 227
Nightingale, Florence, 272
Nurse practitioner, 264–265

O

Oral glucose tolerance test, 114–115
Orlistat, 164–165

P

Paleo diet, 154–155; 277
Pasteur, Louis, 273
Patch (nicotine), 189
Patient Health Questionnaire (PAR-Q 2), 289
Peer pressure , 184

Pembrokeshire Proverb, 55
Personal stories
        -Baseball, 238–239
        -Blood Pressure, 100–101
        -Depression, 250–251
        -Diabetes, 107
        -Exercise, 225–226
        -Farmer, 53
        -Gynecologist, 249
        -Memory, 288
        -Motivational Interviewing, 299–300
        -Choking, 160
        -Red Velvet Cake, 68
        -Restaurant, 142–143
        -Risk taking, 243–244
Phone a friend, 235–236
Physical activity
        -Air pollution, 219
        -Benefits, 202–204
        -Cold weather, 217
        -Current recommendations, 205–206
        -High altitudes, 217–219
        -Hot weather, 215–217
        -Weight, 212–213; 219
Physician assistant, 265
Physician/doctor, 266
Pit falls to changing, 150-151
Plaque build-up, 31-35
Polyunsaturated fats (oils), 69
Portion
        -Control, 138–143
Popular diets, 153–158
Prayer/meditation stress reduction, 236
Pre-diabetes, 114; 119

Pre-hypertension, 81–82
Pregnancy induced hypertension, 85
Preventive Cardiovascular Nurses Association, 303
Primary hypertension, 84–85
Progressive relaxation, 235
Pros versus cons, 244–245; 294
Provider barriers, 254–255
Psychological barrier, 131–138; 248–251; 255

Q

Quality of life, 251; 303–305
Quitting tips, 196; 328
Quotes
    -Agaida Shoshone Tribal Woman, 285
    -*Bible*, Proverbs 29:11, 239
    -Carnegie, Dale, 19
    -Ford, Henry, 241
    -Fuller, Thomson, 306
    -Lovecraft, H. P., 37
    -Niebuhr, Reinhold, 227
    -Roosevelt, Eleanor, 197
    -Skinner, James, 202–203
    -Stanley, Edward, 199
    -Twain, Mark, 169
    -Voltaire, 261
    -Wansink, Brian, 15–16; 125

R

Radiation exposure, 49
Randomized control trial, 275–277
Rapport, 297–298
Red Velvet Cake story, 68

Registered nurse, 263–264

Relaxation, 235

Research, 271–284

Restaurant industry, 142–143

Risk calculator, 42-44; 73-74

Road rage, 236–237

Roosevelt, Eleanor, 197

S

Salt/sodium, 90–93

Sample size, 276–277

Saturated fat article, 278–279

Saturated fats, 62–64

Screening recommendations, 268–270

Secondary hypertension, 85

Secondhand smoke, 180–182

Self-efficacy, 245–246; 294–295; 298

Semmelweis, Ignaz, 272

Side effects from medications, 256; 301–302

Simple Count Method, 42–43

Size difference in research, 276–277

Skinner, James, 202–203

Smoking, 32; 94; 169–198

Smoking quitting strategies, 186; 328

Smokeless tobacco, 178; 182–183; 194–196

Smoking quitting timeline, 186

Snacks, 149

Snow, John, 273–274

Social smoking, 175

Social support, 248–249

South Beach Diet, 155–156

Stages of change, 242–247; 292–296

Stale Movie Popcorn study, 131–132

Stanley, Edward, 199
Starvation diets, 158
Statins, 74–76
Stimulant, 94–96; 184
Stress, 96; 227–239
        -Harm of stress, 229–230
        -Physical exercise and stress, 234
        -Stressors, 230–233; 236–239
Stress testing, 44–45
Stone, Sharon, 52
Stroke
        -Complications, 30–31
        -Symptoms, 27–29; 215
        -Treatment, 29–30
Super Bowl Chicken Wing study, 133–134
Symptoms
        -Diabetes, 113–115
        -Heart attack, 22–23; 213–214
        -Stroke, 27-29; 215

T

Taking first baby steps, 245–246; 294
Talk test, 209–210
Target heart rates, 207–209; 239
Thiazide drugs, 98–99
Thirdhand smoke, 182
Thomson, Virgil, 259
Time out, 234
Tips for taking medication, 258; 301–302
Tobacco, 173
Top 10 weight loss strategies, 166
Total cholesterol, 59

Tourniquet example, 20–21
Trans-fats, 66–68
Triglycerides, 59–60
Twain, Mark, 169
Type 1/Type 2 diabetes, 105–111

U

V

Varencline (Chantix), 192–193
VLDL cholesterol, 58
Voltaire, 261

W

Waist circumference, 129–130
Walking, 223
Wansink studies
 -Bottomless Soup Bowl, 133
 -Comfort Foods, 135–136
 -Ice Cream Social, 132
 -Illusion of Size, 136–137
 -Hershey Kisses, 134–135
 -M&M's Color, 134
 -Stale Movie Popcorn, 131–132
 -Super Bowl Wings, 133–134
 -Wine Connoisseurs study, 133
Warm-ups, 206–207
Web information, 282

Weight management, 94; 108–109; 125–167; 191; 219
    -Categories, 127–129
    -Training, 212–213
    -Weight Watchers, 157
White coat syndrome, 86; 100–101
Wooden, John, 103; 271
Wound healing (diabetes), 113

X, Y and Z

Zyban (bupropion), 191–192

CPSIA information can be obtained
at www.ICGtesting.com
Printed in the USA
LVOW01s1022041216
515736LV00010B/675/P